'I was introduced to Charmaine D'Souza and the benefits of naturopathy by a friend who vouched for its positive effects on our health. I believe in the holistic approach of healthy living as my philosophy is 'Love Yourself'. The best way to treat all root causes and symptoms of any illness even as common as cough, cold, headache, fatigue, and flu is available easily in our kitchen in its most unadulterated form and Charmaine's naturopathy remedies introduced me to that.

I love it as it is a totally natural and drug-free treatment method, safe and effective for both adults and children. And now that it is a regular part of my life, I truly recommend it to all. Charmaine is an ever-smiling, easily accessible angel ready with her list of magical mixes and I am happy to have found her. Wishing her loads of success in all she does always'—Bipasha Basu, Actor

'Charmaine D'Souza is a powerhouse of naturopathy'—Padmini Kolhapure, Actor

'Charmaine is a magician. Her scientific approach in treating every morsel of food one eats towards healing an ailment or losing weight works wonders. Results are seen within two days of following the diet by even around 80 per cent. She even has a solution to a cheat meal! I am thankful to her for keeping me and my family healthy'—Kavita Barjatya, Director, Film and TV Producer, Rajshri Productions (P) Ltd

'Being a mum to two little boys who are so full of energy, I have to constantly be at my fittest best. I started Charmaine's programme even before the birth of my second son and I'm glad to say I have been able to stay healthy and active despite my hectic schedule. I want to continue Charmaine's magical powders as not only do they help in weight loss but also with overall detoxification and cleansing of the system'—Kaykasshan A Patel, Actor

'We always believed in the benefit of natural elements, but discovered the magic of herbs and spices when we met Charmaine two years back in Mumbai. The mix prescribed is now one vital part of our life and keeps us happy and healthy in more ways than one. Thank you, Charmaine.'—Promita and Sanjay Thapar, CEO, Living Media–Hearst Corp Joint Venture

'I have been interacting with Charmaine for the last 10 years. I have found her diet extremely effective—it keeps my body light and energetic through the day. She is a wonderful person and has a remedy for all health matters' —Rajesh Jaggi, Partner, Everstone Capital

'We live in a superfast, advanced environment and have surrendered to artificial methods of survival with multiple side effects. It is high time we return to our traditional Indian methods of treatment. This is exactly what Charmaine does. She guides us to regain the natural immune system of the body so that we are able to fight disease through common herbs and spices found in our very own kitchen. I congratulate Charmaine D'Souza for her in-depth and extensive study on Indian herbs. I recommend her books to all those who are interested in a healthy body and long life. Wishing all the readers great health in abundance'—Dr Atta F Khatri, Family Physician

'Coming from a healthcare empire, it is easy for me to pop pills any time, but Charmaine has changed my outlook. I go to her book *Kitchen Clinic* for remedies before popping that paracetamol for common illness. I also recommend her water therapies to all our gym members'—Upasna Kamineni, Vice President, Apollo Philanthropy and Managing Director, Apollo Life, Hyderabad

'Meeting Charmaine was just by chance. I read her book *Kitchen Clinic* and threw the desire out into the universe—'I want Charmaine to take care of my health'. I am a practising homeopath from Mumbai. Nature cure and natural remedies have always attracted me. Trust me, I don't take to homeopath medicines very easily.

In 2013, my metabolism slowed down, I lost lateral one-third of my eyebrows and on investigation, my thyroid hormones were low. According to conventional medicine, I was advised thyronorm, but I refused to give in. I contacted Charmaine and expressed my desire to put myself on the road to recovery with the help of her treatment. Charmaine checked my reports thoroughly and after a good history taking, whispered a quick prayer and immediately penned down a few herbs and spices on paper. What I appreciate about her approach is transparency. My health was literally in my hands! I had a doubt to begin with but I had no choice. I had to go with this treatment as I was against taking hormone replacement.

Charmaine opened doors of knowledge to many subjects just by incorporating herbs and spices and their powders in my diet. I was feeling much more energetic and good, but I still had a doubt as to whether these things would help improve my hormone levels. My doubts and anxiety were relieved at the end of two-and-a-half months, when I re-tested for the hormone. I was relieved to see the hormone levels more towards normal—I cannot speak of it enough! These levels have remained in the normal range even after I stopped regular treatment. I only have to take an on-and-off dose of the powder I prepare by myself in my kitchen.

What I appreciate about Charmaine is that she guides us to handle our bodies all by ourselves, with no apprehension. I can only sum up: Charmaine is helping mankind to go closer to their roots, yes, closer to Mother Nature'—Dr Payal Advani, BHMS, Mumbai; Access Consciousness Practitioner, Australia; and Mindscape Healer, Singapore

'I call Charmaine my earth angel. In spite of not having a genetic history or any serious health problems, my erratic work schedule had affected my overall health and well-being. Allopathy could not cure my deficiencies or take care of the root cause of my hormonal imbalance which had altered my personality. Charmaine helped me get back my energy levels and restore my imbalances which were causing an upheaval in my whole system. I can actually feel and see the dramatic changes as I keep following her instructions as she fine-tunes my health back to its ideal condition. Her genuine interest and enthusiasm in me and all her clients getting well is touching and I have absolute faith that I will achieve all my health parameters with her gentle, professional, and consistent guidance. She is kind, discreet, and compassionate and has a magic touch. I have absolute faith that not just me but anyone who takes her assistance will always go back with positive results. In complete gratitude of a miracle called Charmaine and of her inspiring work'—Kavita Kapoor, Media Professional; Grooming, Etiquette and Communications Consultant; and Personal Development Coach

'Charmaine has a natural gift of understanding the human body and using natural ingredients in balancing the body. She has been helping many of my family members and me to effectively address and heal different day-to-day ailments and even more complex ones. I am glad and grateful to have met Charmaine'—Madhulika and Abhay Choksi, Director, Hindustan Platinum

'Charmaine's organic and holistic process and easy-to-prepare kitchen remedies have done wonders for me by helping bring down my blood pressure, stabilize my diabetes and control water retention. She is a great listener and an astute therapist who tries to patiently understand every individual's needs, body type, and problems before designing their treatment. I am thankful for her help and wish her the very best'—Shashikant Choksi, Managing Director, Hindustan Platinum

'Charmaine has been helping us with our diet plans and spice mixes for many years. This has made us feel healthier, more energetic, and fit. The fact that the ingredients for the spice mix come from our own kitchen and that the spice mix is also made in our kitchen adds to the appeal of her nutrition programme. Health=Happiness=Charmaine D'Souza'—Naveen Agarwal, Chairman, Sesa Sterlite Limited, Chairman, Cairn India Limited, and Deputy Executive Chairman, Vedanta Resources Plc

'Proper dietary advice before conception, during pregnancy, after birth and later at every stage of adulthood is an essential part of healthy living. We need more and more events to be held on nutrition science to bring about increased dietary awareness. Charmaine's dietary advice, based on her profound study of nutrition science, makes her therapy even more effective than prescribed medicines. It is remarkable that she has found emerging areas in the ever-increasing pressure on global food systems and dietary habits. Her efforts in sharing her knowledge in her books for the health and wellness of the common man are commendable'—Subodh Sapre, President, Dhanwantari Hospital, and VP and Trustee, The Modern School, Mumbai

'Charmaine has turned our health around. Her holistic approach and kind manner has helped us sustain the programme on which she has put us. We credit our well-being to her and wish her more success in the future'—Rupal and Vishad Mafatlal, Vice Chairman, Arvind Mafatlal Group

'I have been following Charmaine's prescribed course of spice mixes since the past two years. I have had amazing results with my diabetes management. Despite my hectic work schedule, I have been able to control my blood sugars well. I just follow her prescribed dosage of spice mix. The powder which is made in my kitchen has miraculous healing and rejuvenating power. She has been able to treat many of my ailments as well as those of my family members.

I am glad to have been introduced to her line of treatment. May God bless her so that she continues this journey to help mankind maintain health and fitness'—Ripudaman Gupta, Tech Director, Kundan Industries Ltd

'Charmaine's simple yet extremely effective remedies use ingredients which are found in our kitchen and transform them into a wonderful and energizing mixture. Charmaine is a genuine person who has made a difference to my well-being! Now, not a day goes by when I don't have her mixtures'—Shalini Jalan, Director, Neo Foods Pvt. Ltd

'Charmaine's mixes have worked fundamentally in keeping me in the pink of health over the past few years. I recommend her all the way'—Kanika Agarwal, Bhoruka Group

'I was fortunate to come across Charmaine when I needed help with my health. My energy levels were very low, even though I felt I was doing everything correctly. As I tend to favour all things natural, Charmaine's holistic approach to health and healing was just what I was looking for. The therapeutic waters and spice mixes have definitely helped improve my energy levels. Her advice is easy to follow and she is always accessible, should you need her. I continue to follow Charmaine's programme to help obtain optimal health'—Jayshree Babani, Perfect Vision, Dubai

'When a mutual friend graciously introduced me to Charmaine, her reputation as a naturopath nutritionist had already preceded her. Even so, the results I got in just a couple of months were extraordinary. I couldn't believe that simple homemade powders of spices and herbs could work such wonders. My overall health has improved vastly and multiple issues have all been taken care of successfully. It is very impressive. She studies each individual case with such dedication and commitment, putting her heart and soul into it, that I believe that she is blessed by God's grace. Her knowledge of nutrition and spices is nothing short of amazing. She is a panacea of wellness. I sincerely urge others to take advantage of her knowledge which she has graciously shared through her books. She is God's gift to our community and deserves all the recognition possible'—Vincent Mathias, Founder Chairman, Christian Chamber of Commerce and Industry, Mumbai

'Charmaine knows all the one-of-a-kind, secret, natural, innovative remedies that can easily be incorporated into one's daily life. Completely different from what you would expect! Makes you feel naturally fit and healthy'—Viveka Narang, Director, Narang Group

'For more than one year, we have been taking Charmaine's herbal mix which we make in our kitchen. With her simple and easy-to-use remedies, she has brought about a very positive change in our health. It has helped us in boosting our immunity, better digestion, good sleep, and good general health'—Darshana and Suresh Gupta, Managing Director, Radiant Luxury Developers Pvt. Ltd

'Charmaine's therapeutic method has been the best thing that I have experienced to improve my health. It is organic and natural and is made by my staff in my kitchen. My cholesterol, diabetes, and the rest of my blood profile has been well taken care of, despite my inability to fully comply with the regimen because of me work. For this, I am ever grateful to her'—Uma Agarwal, Bhoruka Gases

'Over the past 20 years, at different times of medical need, I've benefited from complete cures based on Charmaine's natural and holistic approach to nutrition. Most recently, her prescribed regimen normalized my diabetic fathers HbA1c levels improving his quality of life. My faith in Charmaine continues to grow every day'—Ritika Jain Ghai, Interior Designer, New York

'Charmaine is blessed with a gift—a gift to cure with kitchen herbs. She is totally committed, passionate and works for the wellbeing of the client. She has made a big difference to our lives—Durga Raheja, Mumbai

'Charmaine's treatments are individually geared and very simple to follow. She recommends using natural spices and herbs for overall health benefits. Excellent'—Miloni Mafatlal, Health Addict, Zurich

'Since working with Charmaine and following the nutritional advice, I have noticed that my blood sugar has been lower at any time of the day and also the glycosylated sugars over three months have come down. The micronutrients and other nutrients that are in the various mixes have improved my overall health and energy levels. I really appreciate the discipline it has brought into my life'—A well wisher, Gujarat

BLOOD SUGAR & SPICE

Living with DIABETES

CHARMAINE D'SOUZA

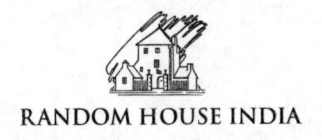

RANDOM HOUSE INDIA

Published by Random House India in 2014
1

Copyright © Charmaine D'Souza 2014

Random House Publishers India Pvt Ltd
7th Floor, Infinity Tower C, DLF Cyber City
Gurgaon – 122002
Haryana

Random House Group Limited
20 Vauxhall Bridge Road
London SW1V 2SA
United Kingdom

978 81 8400 593 6

This book is sold subject to the condition that it shall not, by way of trade or otherwise, be lent, resold, hired out, or otherwise circulated without the publisher's prior consent in any form of binding or cover other than that in which it is published and without a similar condition including this condition being imposed on the subsequent purchaser.

Typeset in Adobe Garamond Pro by R. Ajith Kumar

Printed and bound in India by Replika Press Private Limited

A PENGUIN RANDOM HOUSE COMPANY

*To my husband Savio and my daughters
Charylene and Savylene*

Also by Charmaine D'Souza

Kitchen Clinic

Contents

Foreword by Naresh Goyal — xiii
Introduction — xv

I: EXPLAINING DIABETES — 1

1. What is Diabetes? — 5
2. The Complications of Diabetes — 31
3. Myths and FAQs — 44

II: MANAGING DIABETES — 55

4. Controlling Diabetes with Allopathic Medication — 59
5. Controlling Diabetes with Diet — 70
6. Controlling Diabetes with Herbs, Spices, and Supplements — 112
7. Healthy Recipes — 125
8. The Way Forward — 145
9. A Dictionary for Diabetics — 151

Appendix A: Cheating Out — 201
Appendix B: Your Health Record Chart — 203
Acknowledgements — 213
A Note on the Author — 217

Foreword

Health is our greatest asset. Good health leads to success at work with increased efficiency and a great family life with prosperity and happiness. The more you have of good health, the more you have of these. Alarmingly, as employers, we see increasingly rising costs of healthcare of our employees, with increased susceptibility to heart disease, cancer, diabetes, obesity, chronic aches and pains, kidney ailments, and other such stress-related conditions with their adverse impact on overall staff welfare.

Good health and general well-being affect every aspect of an individual's life. As Chairman of Jet Airways, my role requires me to optimize the welfare of my staff and the market share and profitability of my company continuously. It is a complex role, entailing constant travel at odd hours cross-country and across continents and time zones, in a punishing schedule that includes erratic waking, sleep, and eating hours. These soon began to affect my health. I felt my vitality and life quality visibly diminish and so I made an internal decision to correct this unhealthy situation for the sake of my family, my colleagues, and my company.

When I first met Charmaine, she was already helping my family members and some of my employees stay fit and healthy. Encouraged by my wife with whom I had shared my personal decision, I decided to try out Charmaine's 'Good Health

Always' programme. She explained to me that even though I had access to the finest medical care, my health still required my own personal attention and effort. Among other measures, she formulated a healthy eating pattern for me to enable me to stay fit and energetic and continue to enjoy the work that I do, as well as, hopefully, set an example for my team.

Charmaine's dedication, commitment, and ability to heal with the use of simple kitchen herbs and spices are the bedrock of her success. In this book, and in her earlier work, Charmaine has made the concepts of naturopathy more accessible to the lay person. Her simple DIY approach allows people with health issues, but without extensive medical knowledge, to successfully help themselves. Diabetes is a widespread disease and a book on diabetes which laymen can read and understand is very relevant in today's stressful times. *Blood Sugar and Spice: Living with Diabetes* considers the person suffering from the disease in the context of their family members rather than just having a medical viewpoint.

From my personal experience, I would urge you to read, understand, and follow the advice that Charmaine gives in her book, though first do discuss it with your medical practitioner. I am sure that it will improve your health and change your life for the better. I would advise the reader to use the book as a tool to achieve the level of health and well-being that will make for sound health and overall happiness. After reading this book, I hope you are as inspired as I am to realize how important good health is in enjoying every aspect of our lives.

I am sure the book will be tremendously appreciated and I wish Charmaine all the best in her future endeavours.

Naresh Goyal
Chairman, Jet Airways

Introduction

More than 24 years ago, I walked into my therapeutic dietetic board practical examination and pulled out a chit for my topic. My heart sank. My chit read 'Plan an 1800-calorie diet for a Type 2 diabetic patient with high blood pressure'. Even though I knew I would be able to do a good job, having pored over numerous calorie sheets and textbooks the previous night, the external examiner for this practical examination was Dr G.D. Koppikar, well known in the dietetic field as a meticulous taskmaster, someone who could scare even the most confident of dietetic students. More importantly, Dr Koppikar was the Chief Dietician of S.L. Raheja Hospital, Mumbai, which at that time was exclusively for diabetic patients. The diet planning and food preparation part of the practical went off well, or so I thought! I vividly remember the viva: Dr Koppikar at her sternest best peering at my diet sheet, at the meal I had prepared and grilling me for more than 20 minutes, which to me seemed like over two hours. I finished, cleared my stuff from the table, and left the room, sure that I had goofed up. An hour later she called for me once again; scary thoughts ran through my mind. My hands shook, my heart was beating out of my chest. I felt that I had probably goofed up so badly that she wanted to question me once again, just to give me a passing grade. Instead I heard her ask if I would like to do an internship at her hospital … since I had done so well! Later she told me that she felt I had potential and hence offered me the double internship even though she knew I would first have to complete my compulsory internship at KEM Hospital, Mumbai.

I learned a lot during that year under Dr Koppikar's tutelage. I learned how to deal with diabetics who had various health complications, how to handle their relatives, how to deal with hospital staff, and, most importantly, how to empathize and not sympathize with the patients in order to get them to follow dietary instructions so that their health would improve. Hospital dieticians have a tough job, trying their best to get OPD patients to follow instructions while they themselves have to adhere to what the patients' doctor has ordered/prescribed. So if the doctor is a strict vegetarian and feels that all his patients should follow vegetarianism, the dietician will be pulled up if she allows the patient an occasional serving of chicken. Try telling a Parsi or Catholic diabetic patient to stop eating non-vegetarian food—he/she will look at you as though you have lost it! Often I would sit in the OPD which was on the ground floor of the hospital, prescribe a diet according to hospital rules and guidelines, and watch in horror as the same patient with uncontrolled diabetes would walk right out of the hospital gate with his blood reports, doctor's prescription, and diet sheet all neatly filed and happily tuck into a plateful of goodies that the corner sev-puri wallah was dishing out, followed by a mound of creamy, cloyingly sweet kulfi with rabdi! My colleagues and I would then often bet on how soon we would see that patient admitted in the general ward of the hospital or, God forbid, in the ICU.

With hospitalized patients, compliance was always easier

because the patient only had access to what was served to them at mealtimes—unless a 'kind' relative or friend sneaked in some banned goodies. The ones who did not have access to this would grumble every time we went on ward rounds. They were not happy with the food, the medication, the staff, the room, the other patients, the relatives, the hospital clothes, and so on and so forth. We gave each of them a patient hearing because we could feel their pain and knew that the root cause of their unhappiness was the fact that they were unable to maintain a control on their blood glucose levels. This is probably where I learned to 'listen' to what they were not saying aloud. Also, most of them were scared because uncontrolled diabetes brought on a host of complications and topping the hospital list were gangrene and lower limb amputation.

Later, I also started teaching nutrition and dietetics at Jaslok Hospital, Mumbai and at a number of catering colleges in the city.

In my first book, *Kitchen Clinic*, I said that I am humbled by the faith people have in me, that it overwhelms me and sometimes even scares me. It is this implicit faith that my clients have in me that eggs me on to do the best I possibly can to help them. They keep coming back to me because they see results. The 'holistic' approach I prescribe in my **Good Health Always** programme considers the whole person and how he/she interacts with his/her environment. My clients are motivated not just by the number of kilograms they lose, but by how good they feel when they find reserves of energy and enthusiasm for life, how well they sleep at night, how much calmer they are, and, most importantly, by the knowledge that their health is truly in their hands. It goes without saying that their improved blood glucose levels, lipid profile, renal profile, blood pressure reading, etc. are further and, for me, the 'most important' proof that this programme works! **The main objective of the programme is the prevention of illness or the cure of ailments, with the use of kitchen herbs and spices so that the body maintains and heals itself.**

Kitchen Clinic was very well appreciated and got very good reviews. The book reviews, emails, calls, and messages from readers from all parts of the country and also from abroad have served to further overwhelm me. People I have never met or spoken to have written in to say how thankful they are to me for sharing my knowledge on naturopathy. How simple tips like the one on the therapeutic celery water have helped them bring down their blood pressure and consequently made their doctors confidently decrease the dosage of their medication. For this and other blessings, I am truly grateful to God.

Over the last 24 years of my dietetic practice, I have learned to tell my patients to 'Listen to your body and follow its lead'. By doing this we can learn how to protect our body, make it strong and disease-free, and, most of all, enjoy good health … always! This is precisely what this book, on dealing with diabetes, is all about. It has information on all that you need to know once you, or a family member, or a friend has been diagnosed with the condition. It seeks to give you a better understanding of what this endocrine condition is all about, how to cope with it, the blood tests you should do to monitor your blood glucose levels and other health parameters, the foods you should eat and the ones you should avoid in order to have a tight control over your blood glucose levels … how to take charge of your own health.

This is the kind of book I wish I had as a child, when my father was diagnosed with diabetes. I spent most of my childhood watching him try various methods, pills, and potions to keep his blood glucose levels under control. Ultimately he succumbed to cancer.

We spend most of our life ill-treating our body, not realizing that our body will not last forever, that it is the only one we will ever have, at least in this lifetime! We deprive our body of sleep because of our crazy work schedules and even crazier partying. We deprive our body of food just to fit into skinny jeans or to get down to 'size zero', conveniently forgetting that the epitome of size zero is now promoting 'healthy eating'. After years of abuse we wonder why our organs stop functioning well. We wonder why insulin resistance sets in, why our blood pressure rises even though we go on 'salt-free days', why our weight increases, why our cholesterol levels increase even though we limit our intake of fried food. Then comes the dreaded diagnosis of diabetes, hypertension, obesity, hypercholesterolemia, etc., all leading to Syndrome X. This is a very crucial time, a time when we need to map out possible treatment strategies with the help of a 'healthcare team'.

The healthcare team includes all the people who work with you to help manage your diabetes: your endocrinologist or diabetes doctor, cardiologist or heart doctor, nephrologist or kidney doctor, podiatrist or foot doctor, ophthalmologist or eye doctor, dentist, nutritionist or dietician, hospital nurse, diabetes educator and counsellor, physiotherapist, exercise strategist, community health worker, and even your health coach. You can use this book to keep some records about your health. At the end of this book there are forms to write down details about your health and your general concerns. Please photocopy these pages and fill in the details of your blood glucose levels, etc.

so that you can take them with you whenever you visit your healthcare team. Do ensure that you go over these records frequently with your healthcare team. It also makes it easier for your doctor to help you. Being in charge and keeping track of your health is one of the ways you can work together with your healthcare team to control your diabetes.

It is important to write down the names and telephone numbers of each and every member of your healthcare team. Keep in touch with your healthcare team members regularly by way of a phone call, text message, email or even a WhatsApp message. This way, they will also be concerned when they do not hear from you for a long period of time. Make it a regular practice to jot down questions and other points you want to remember when you speak to or visit the team members.

Read the section on diabetic diets carefully. It will give you an idea of what your carbohydrate, protein, fat, water, vitamin, and mineral intake should be, as well as your intake of caffeine, artificial sweeteners, alcohol, etc. Chapter 6, 'Controlling Diabetes with Herbs, Spices, and Supplements', is a chapter that is very dear to me. Make sure you read this chapter thoroughly and discuss with your healthcare practitioner before you start incorporating some of these aforementioned herbs and spices in your daily diet. Keep a record of your blood glucose levels once you start using the herbs and spices. This will help you determine how much you have benefited from them, in your quest for keeping a tight control over your blood glucose levels and also for preventing diabetes-related complications.

Healthy food has to also taste good in order for it to do good for our body. It supports the integrity of our body, nurtures it, and keeps us fit. So by popular demand, I have also incorporated some recipes tested in our 'Good Health Always' kitchen, which you can easily try out at home. Feedback at goodhealthalways@outlook.com is most welcome and will be highly appreciated, especially if you keep a record of your blood glucose levels after preparing and consuming one of the dishes mentioned in this recipe section. So go ahead and try some of these recipes that are targeted towards helping you maintain good health ... always!

If you really love yourself and want to enjoy the very best of physical and mental health, this book will guide you every step of the way and help you make that happen. There is absolutely nothing more empowering than being in control of decisions regarding your health. Good health is God's greatest blessing. So stay blessed with good health ... always!

Charmaine D'Souza
August 2014, Mumbai

I

Explaining Diabetes

Eating too much sugar *does not* give you diabetes—you have your genes and your lifestyle to thank for that—but when you have diabetes mellitus it is not advisable to eat too much sugar or any sugar at all, depending on your level of blood sugar control. This is easier said than done given that we live in a world where newer and yummier desserts are being dished out by top chefs everywhere. We also live in a country where ending every meal on a sweet note is the norm and every festival and announcement of 'good news' is celebrated with oodles of mithai and sweetmeats of all kinds. In my 24 years of practice I have often received 'thank-yous' from diabetics who use my therapeutic spice-mix recipes and are thereby better able to control their blood sugar levels. This is a very rewarding as well as humbling experience because it was diabetes that first inspired me to research into and create different therapeutic spice-mix recipes to help diabetics live with the disease. I started my career at the S.L. Raheja Hospital which, in the early 1990s, catered solely to diabetic patients and those with complications arising from uncontrolled diabetes. My father had diabetes and so do a number of my friends and relatives; even my young daughters have schoolmates with juvenile diabetes. In fact, whenever I describe the work I do as a nutritionist 'everyone' seems to know someone with this metabolic disease. This comes as no surprise given the alarming rate at which diabetes is growing. Even more alarming is the fact that there are millions of people who have diabetes and are not even aware of it. Also, there are so many people who have pre-diabetes, a condition where the person's blood sugar levels are higher than normal but not high enough to warrant diabetic medication. Diabetes mellitus is one of the most problematic diseases of today.

More than 112,000 children in India have Type 1 diabetes. 14 November is celebrated as World Diabetes Day (WDD). Isn't it ironic that we Indians also celebrate Children's Day on 14 November, the birthday of Pandit Jawaharlal Nehru? India has the dubious distinction of being the diabetes capital of the world. As of 2011, more than 61 million Indians have been diagnosed with diabetes according to the International Diabetes Federation (IDF). Figures now indicate that if proper action against the disease is not taken quickly, there will be 10 million new cases diagnosed every year, so that by 2030 there will be 552 million diabetic people worldwide. What is even more alarming is that there are millions of people who are blissfully unaware that they have this deadly disease. Diabetes can be controlled with diet, exercise, and medication. When it is well managed, many of the risks associated with this disease are reduced. However, if diabetes is poorly managed, or more alarmingly, not diagnosed, it can have a devastating impact on the quality and length of the patient's life.

1
What is Diabetes?

Diabetes mellitus (DM) is a group of metabolic diseases in which the blood sugar of a person is higher than normal. The name diabetes mellitus comes from two Greek words: 'diabetes' meaning 'siphon' and 'mellitus' meaning 'honey'. It describes a condition in which blood glucose cannot be absorbed properly. The term 'blood sugar' always refers to the glucose circulating in the blood, although small amounts of other sugars may also be present in the blood stream for short periods of time. Abnormally high blood sugar levels can cause several short-term and long-term complications. High blood sugar causes frequent urination (polyurea) as well as an increase in thirst (polydipsia) and hunger (polyphagia) that is much more than normal. If the blood glucose levels get elevated, the kidneys are not able to filter all the glucose. Some of this extra glucose escapes or spills out into the urine. The extra glucose thickens the urine and draws in extra water to help it flow through the kidneys. This in turn causes the bladder to fill up more easily and, as a result, the patient with uncontrolled diabetes needs to urinate copiously and very frequently (polyurea). Due to this excessive urination the body gets dehydrated, leading to increased thirst (polydipsia). Dehydration can lead to constipation and passing of hard stools. Our bodies acquire energy from glucose and a diabetic, being unable to access blood glucose, will lack energy and will be tired or lethargic through the day. Body cells and tissues will break down to replace this energy, causing dramatic weight loss without any diet regimen. This unexplained weight loss can be attributed to untreated diabetes. If left untreated, diabetes may cause many serious complications like diabetic ketoacidosis, coma, heart disease, kidney failure, amputation of the lower limbs, and damage to the eyes. In some diabetics, the excess glucose which is circulating in the blood stream can cause it to thicken, leading to difficulty in focusing and blurry vision. Due to the elevations in blood sugar, the functioning of the immune system can also get impaired, making a diabetic susceptible to many infections like urinary tract infections, skin rashes, and eruptions as well as upper respiratory infections. Nerve functioning can also get impaired resulting in tingling, tenderness, pins and needles, burning, lack of sensation, and numbness of the palms of the hands and the soles of the feet.

Diabetes insipidus (DI) is a metabolic condition whose symptoms include excessive thirst (polydipsia) and the passing of copious amounts of diluted urine (polyuria). Diabetes insipidus comes from the Latin word 'inspidus' meaning 'insipid' or 'lacking taste' because DI is not characterized by glycosuria. It may be caused due to a deficiency of the antidiuretic hormone (ADH) or by the insensitivity of the kidneys to ADH. There is a small percentage of people with diabetes whose condition is due to DI and not due to DM. Even though they share a common name, DM and DI are totally separate conditions caused by unrelated mechanisms. It is very important to note that the urine of a patient with DI does not contain sugar while that of a DM patient contains it due to the high amount of blood sugar which ultimately leaks out into the urine.

The carbohydrate glucose is a form of sugar that is the main source of fuel needed to energize the body. When we eat a meal comprising carbohydrates like rice, wheat, jowar, bajra, ragi, potatoes, sweet potato, yam, tapioca, beans, sugary desserts, etc., we absorb glucose from these foods. The chewing of food in the mouth allows the enzymes present in our saliva to start breaking down these foods and this process of digestion continues in the stomach. This partially digested food then goes into the small intestine where the process of digestion continues and the food breaks down into very small particles including those of glucose. Glucose is then absorbed into the bloodstream from where it moves into the liver where it is stored for future use or burned up to provide us with the energy needed to do work.

Several hormones contribute to abnormal blood sugar levels. The main problem is an imbalance between the supply and demand for insulin. Insulin is a peptide hormone that is produced by the beta cells of the islets of Langerhans in the pancreas. Insulin is needed to regulate both carbohydrate as well as fat metabolism in the body. Insulin causes skeletal muscle cells as well as cells of fat tissue to absorb glucose from the blood. When we eat carbohydrate-rich food like rice, roti, pasta, starchy vegetables like potato, yam, etc. as well as desserts, the carbohydrates are converted into glucose and it is this glucose which releases energy for us to do work. If insulin is not secreted in sufficient amounts, this glucose circulates in the bloodstream rather than being taken to the different cells. Diabetes mellitus can result when there is a failure in the control of serum insulin levels. Therefore, insulin has to be used to treat some forms of diabetes. Insulin may be endogenous (made within one's body) or exogenous (administered via an injection into subcutaneous tissue). Deficiency of insulin results in hyperglycemia (high blood sugar) while too much of insulin circulating in the system results in hypoglycemia (low blood sugar). Both these conditions can be potentially dangerous to a diabetic patient. Some patients can have a condition called insulin resistance whereby their blood sugar levels continue to be abnormally high despite having a high level of circulating insulin.

Despite medical advancement and years of research by healthcare professionals and pharmaceutical companies, there has been no breakthrough in finding a cure for this disease. There is no information on why the pancreas suddenly stops producing insulin in people with Type 1 diabetes. Some people have a genetic predisposition to diabetes so if there is a history of diabetes in your family, do make sure that you regularly get your blood sugar level tested and make appropriate lifestyle changes. In some cases a viral disease can alter your immune system and weaken it. As a result, the beta cells of the islets of Langerhans of the pancreas get destroyed and hence cannot produce insulin. Type 2 diabetes is often associated with a genetic predisposition and can be linked with obesity. It is scary to see the growing number of young children with Type 2 diabetes due to an unhealthy lifestyle. Gestational diabetes or glucose intolerance during pregnancy sometimes disappears after the birth of the baby but predisposes the mother to diabetes during later pregnancies and also later on in life. Overactivity of the thyroid gland can also contribute to the incidence of diabetes mellitus, as does the long-term use of steroids.

CONDITIONS FREQUENTLY ASSOCIATED WITH CHANGES IN THE BLOOD SUGAR LEVELS

A. The metabolic condition of diabetes mellitus which is of two types: Type 1 and Type 2.
B. Stress-induced hyperglycemia, when the serum blood sugars increase because of severe debilitating accidents and injuries, burns, major surgery like gastrectomy, and heart diseases like myocardial infarction.
C. Infusions of concentrated amounts of glucose that are given through a drip as in the case of Total Parenteral Nutrition (TPN) wherein the patient receives a combination of glucose, amino acids, fats, vitamins, minerals, and water through a drip feed.
D. Food-stimulated or reactive hypoglycemia which is very rare but may occur secondary to gastrectomy where a part or all of the stomach is removed mainly to combat obesity in a morbidly obese patient.
E. Disease-related hypoglycemia: when the blood sugar levels fall because of tumours that produce an additional amount of the hormone insulin or sometimes due to severe liver disease.
F. Drug-related hypoglycemia due to high dosages of hypoglycemic agents like insulin or oral hypoglycemic medications in relation to food intake. Increasing your workout pattern and intensity of the workout can cause dips in the blood sugar level. Similarly, consuming alcohol on an empty stomach or while eating minimally can also cause the blood sugar to fall.

G. Drug-related hyperglycemia in response to steroid therapy as well as the use of diuretics and anti-depressants.

THE VARIOUS SYMPTOMS OF DIABETES

Most readers are aware of the symptoms of diabetes, which although varied are also very obvious in many, if not all, of the cases. Since the disease is so widespread, describe just one or two of the symptoms to a friend and he will immediately ask you to check your blood sugar levels! It is important to understand why these symptoms manifest themselves. Polydipsia or increased thirst, polyphagia or increased hunger, and polyuria or passing of copious amounts of urine are common symptoms that indicate the onset of the disease. Constipation, dramatic weight loss, fatigue, blurring of vision, susceptibility to infections, and the typical pins and needles feeling or burning in the hands or feet because of changes in nerve functioning also characterize diabetes mellitus.

The kidneys play a major role in filtering out glucose. As the blood sugar levels keep increasing in a diabetic patient, the kidneys are unable to filter out all this glucose, which results in some of the glucose escaping out into the urine. The viscosity of the urine increases because of this. More water is now needed to help the urine flow through the kidneys. As more and more water is drawn in, the bladder gets full more quickly than normal resulting in the frequent passing of large amounts of urine. Since more than normal amounts of water are excreted the patient becomes dehydrated and this leads to increased thirst, dry stools, and constipation.

We are well aware that our bodies require energy in order to function properly. This energy is derived from the glucose present in different cells of the body. A diabetic patient cannot get access to the glucose circulating in the bloodstream. Hence he is low on energy and feels tired all the time. Since the primary concern of the body is to provide energy in order to survive, a diabetic patient's body will break down other cells and tissues to get this energy. This causes dramatic weight loss, especially in uncontrolled diabetes.

The excess glucose circulating in a diabetic patient's blood will make it more viscous, resulting in disruptions in eye focus and blurring of vision. Another manifestation of this increased viscosity of blood is a decrease in immunity and the inability to fight infections. Thus a diabetic is susceptible to various infections like those of the urinary tract, upper respiratory tract, and skin. Unfortunately, these infections further increase the patient's blood sugar levels.

In order to stay as healthy as possible a diabetic should strive to maintain his blood sugar levels as near to normal as possible. In order to be able to do this, he should regularly get his blood glucose levels tested. For a more accurate reading the blood should be taken from a vein and not from a finger prick. This is because blood uses up some of the sugar it was originally carrying by the time blood reaches the finger through small blood vessels. Thus the blood glucose reading from a finger prick is generally lower than the venous plasma glucose level.

THE DIAGNOSIS OF DIABETES

Blood Glucose Levels: Normal and Abnormal Values

You may have done a routine blood test or a complete blood count (CBC) and wondered about the significance of your blood sugar readings. The laboratory values used to distinguish hyperglycemia and hypoglycemia vary depending on the choice of serum or whole blood and also the particular method of determination. Hence different laboratories may show different readings of the same blood sample depending on the method of determination that they follow.

In general, when an adult's blood sugar concentration rises above 180 mg of glucose per 100 ml blood, he would be described as diabetic. When the blood sugar level exceeds 160 mg to 180 mg per dl, sugar spills into the urine and the urine test will also be positive for sugar. This condition of sugar in the urine is called glycosuria. Glycosuria is common in patients with uncontrolled diabetes and it can be very easily detected by simple urine tests. A blood glucose concentration of less than about 60 mg per dl indicates hypoglycemia. Urine tests cannot be used to identify hypoglycemia.

The blood glucose levels of a diabetic patient are most meaningful if they are related to time and composition of the most recent meal. Hence most diabetologists encourage their diabetic patients to test their fasting blood sugar (FBS) levels 10–12 hours after dinner and to test their post-prandial or post-meal blood sugar (PPBS) samples exactly two hours after consuming their regular lunch or dinner. The word 'regular' is of significance here because some diabetics eat lesser than normal because they fear a higher sugar reading while there are some patients who eat much more than their normal meal, probably to test the efficacy of the laboratory machine! A random blood sugar (RBS) level is unrelated to food intake and provides useful information only if it falls well outside of normal range. Many diabetologists test the patients' RBS values in their own consulting clinics in order to determine how well their diabetic patient is progressing. A normal fasting blood sugar (FBS) generally lies between about 60 mg and 100 mg glucose per 100 ml blood for adults. A very high FBS is a sign of diabetes mellitus and is usually accompanied by many of the classic symptoms of this deadly disease.

Screening Tests for Diabetes Mellitus

It is not easy to come to terms with the fact that you have diabetes but once a person has been diagnosed with diabetes, it is essential for him to try and maintain his blood sugar levels as near to normal as possible in order to prevent the onset of a myriad medical complications associated with this disease. These complications include heart disease, micro-vascular disease, blindness, and in severe cases, if the disease is left untreated, it may lead to coma and death. For millions of diabetics living around the world, being educated about this metabolic disorder is the first step towards feeling better, being able to cope and living a longer, healthier, and enriched life. Blood sugars are commonly measured by either regular blood glucose testing which gives a reading of the current blood glucose level, or by the glycosylated or glycated hemoglobin level (HbA1C) which gives the clinical practitioner an idea of the patients' average blood glucose levels over the last three months. Another comparatively newer test is to check the diabetic patients' serum fructosamine levels which reflect the changes in blood glucose and the average readings over the recent one to two weeks.

Blood screening tests are very useful for early detection of diabetes mellitus as well as for the abnormalities in the control of blood sugar level. In a screening test, the blood glucose levels are tested at first after the suspected patient has fasted for a minimum of eight hours following a regular carbohydrate-rich meal. The person is then asked to consume a meal containing a minimum of 75–100 gm of carbohydrate. In the Indian context a basic 'thali meal' with roti, rice, dal, vegetables, and dahi would suffice. The blood sugar levels are then tested two hours after the consumption of this meal. If the blood glucose level exceeds a present level, for example 180 mg/dl two hours post-prandial for adults, diabetes mellitus is suspected and further testing may be done.

Further testing for diabetes mellitus includes the glucose tolerance test (GTT), in which the suspected patients' blood glucose level is determined at thirty-minute intervals after the ingestion of about 75–100 gm glucose in the fasting state. GTT is a useful test in the diagnosis of diabetes mellitus or of reactive hypoglycemia. An impaired GTT results in abnormally high levels of blood sugar. This may not always hold true for elderly patients because there is a significant increase in FBS as well as an increase in glucose tolerance (as described by S.S. Fagans and N. Freinkel, 'The Problem of Diabetes Mellitus', in S. S. Fagan [ed.] *Diabetes Mellitus*, Fogarty International Center Series on Preventive Medicine, vol. 4, DHEW pub. no. [MIH]76 584, Bethesda: National Institute of Health, 1976). as we age. Hence healthcare practitioners should be careful while classifying an elderly client as diabetic using criteria that have been developed for younger persons.

The Comparison of Blood Glucose, Fructosamine, and HbA1c Levels

Glucose (mg/dl)	Fructosamine (mmol)	HbA1c (%)
90	212.5	5.0
120	250.0	6.0
150	287.5	7.0
180	325.0	8.0
210	362.5	9.0
240	400.0	10.0
270	437.5	11.0
300	475.0	12.0
330	512.5	13.0
360	550.0	14.0

Source: D. M. Nathan, D. E. Singer, K. Hurxthal, and J. D. Goodson, 'The Clinical Information Value of the Glycosylated Hemoglobin Assay', *The New England Journal of Medicine*, 310 (6): 341–46, February 1984.

How Hormones Play a Significant Role in Altering People's Blood Sugar Levels

In the body of a non-diabetic person, the hormones insulin, glucagon, and somatostatin serve to regulate the blood sugar levels and keep them within the normal range. If for any reason these hormones are unable to fulfil their role in blood sugar metabolism then there will be alterations in the blood sugar levels.

Insulin

Insulin is an anabolic hormone manufactured and stored in the pancreas. Once the blood glucose levels increase typically after the ingestion of a carbohydrate-rich meal, insulin gets released into the bloodstream. It plays a significant role in controlling blood sugar. Insulin increases the uptake of amino acids and glucose by the cells. Once insulin enters the bloodstream it links into insulin receptor sites, causing chemical changes to occur in the cell walls and thereby allowing glucose into the cell. This glucose can now be used to provide the body with energy. Conditions like obesity and diabetes adversely affect these insulin receptor sites, causing alterations in insulin activity as well as alterations in blood sugar levels. The hormone insulin is needed for proper metabolism in the body. Insulin promotes anabolism, an energy-utilizing process of building up of molecules. Some insulin needs to be constantly circulating in the bloodstream in order to prevent excess catabolism from occurring in the different tissues of the body. Catabolism is an energy-releasing process which breaks down complex molecules in the body. When there is lack of proper amounts of insulin circulating in the bloodstream then the person rapidly loses muscle tissue and body fat. By simply altering one's exercise pattern, the efficiency of insulin uptake can be changed. This can also alter the rate at which blood glucose is utilized in the body.

Glucagon

Glucagon is the hormone secreted by the alpha cells of the islets of Langerhans of the pancreas. When the secretion of glucagon gets impaired, there can be changes in the blood sugar levels. Glucagon raises blood sugar levels and thus its effect is the exact opposite of the hormone insulin which lowers the blood sugar levels. The liver stores glycogen to be utilized as and when the body requires energy. Glucagon causes the liver to convert its stores of glycogen into glucose even if the body does not require it at that point of time. This sudden increase in the blood glucose levels in turn causes an increase in the secretion and release of insulin into the bloodstream. Hence it is evident that insulin and glucagon have to team up in order to stabilize the blood sugar levels. However, if the body lacks insulin due to impaired metabolism and if there is an excessive secretion of glucagon, the blood sugars will shoot up even more and hyperglycemia will persist for a longer time. On the other hand, if there is insufficient glucagon secretion, low blood sugar or hypoglycemia will persist for a longer time.

Somatostatin

Somatostatin is the growth hormone–inhibiting hormone that ironically suppresses the production of both insulin as well as glucagon, thereby regulating both these hormones. Somatostatin is a hormone produced and secreted by the delta cells of the islets of Langerhans of the pancreas. It is also produced in the stomach and the intestine.

Others

When some diabetic patients are highly stressed their blood sugar levels increase drastically. The stress could be mental as well as physical. Glucogenic hormones, which are released in response to stress, can be the cause of this increase in the blood glucose levels. These glucogenic hormones (e.g., epinephrine, glucocoriticoids, glucagon, and growth hormones) are sometimes called *insulin-antagonistic* hormones because they impede the action of insulin in lowering the blood sugar levels.

TYPES OF DIABETES MELLITUS

Diabetes mellitus is a group of metabolic diseases characterized by elevations in the blood sugar levels. All patients diagnosed with diabetes lack sufficient amounts of the hormone insulin which is required for normal carbohydrate metabolism. In many cases the deficiency of insulin production is relative and may be overcome without the use of hypoglycemic agents (medications used to bring down the blood sugar level). This can be achieved by making alterations in the patient's lifestyle, increasing exercise, and monitoring the diet.

In order for a diabetologist to treat a patient with DM, it is necessary to classify diabetes mellitus according to type of onset and the need for exogenous insulin.

Insulin-dependent Diabetes Mellitus (IDDM)

The most severe form of DM is also known as Type 1 diabetes or juvenile diabetes (JD). It has a dramatic onset. It is indicated by most of the classic signs of diabetes. Patients with IDDM complain of extreme thirst (polydipsia), excessive hunger (polyphagia) which may be accompanied by unexplained weight loss, and greatly increased frequency of urination (polyuria) especially at night. A laboratory test will show elevated blood sugar levels as well as sugar in the urine (glycosuria). If the condition is not treated effectively and on time then the patient shows dramatic weight loss due to loss of skeletal muscle as well as fat, feels very lethargic and extremely ill, and in a short while develops a serious life-threatening condition called diabetes ketoacidosis (DKA). The patient has to be hospitalized and put on exogenous insulin and fluid electrolyte replacement immediately. After the acute condition of DKA is corrected, the patient is discharged from hospital and chronic treatment requires exogenous insulin and control of diet and exercise for the remainder of the person's life. Since exogenous insulin is required for life, this type of diabetes is often called insulin-dependent diabetes mellitus (IDDM). Despite major advancements made in the medical field it is unfortunate that a complete cure is yet to be found, although research continues.

For some time after the dramatic development of IDDM, patients may occasionally experience a temporary period of partial remission during which the blood sugar levels stay as near as normal. It is during this period that small amounts of insulin are produced by the beta cells of the islets of Langerhans of the pancreas. This period of partial remission is often called the honeymoon period; it is during this time that the recently diagnosed diabetes patient and his family come to terms with the disease and learn how to live with it and deal with it. If immediate insulin and diet treatment follows the diagnosis of juvenile diabetes then some beta-cell activity may be prolonged and the juvenile diabetic may continue to enjoy this honeymoon period for a number of years. Once the blood sugar level is readily controlled by exogenous insulin and a regimented diet and exercise schedule then the IDDM patient is considered stable. Regular monitoring of the blood sugar levels and other blood levels is extremely necessary for the IDDM patient to lead a normal life.

A small percentage of IDDM patients sometimes experience dangerously wide swings in their blood sugar level for no obvious reason. This is despite them adhering to their insulin, diet, and exercise schedules. These low blood sugar (hypoglycemic) and high blood sugar (hyperglycemic) episodes may wreak havoc in their lives, with family members and caregivers often doubting their sincerity in following the stringent line of treatment. This unstable form of IDDM is often called *brittle* diabetes.

Diabetes that is caused due to a pancreatectomy (the surgical removal of the pancreas) has the same characteristics of IDDM.

Devendra Patel, a 52-year-old man suffering from IDDM for the past thirty years, was introduced to me by his wife Parvati, and his daughter-in-law Radha, both of whom I was already helping. He had the scepticism and irritation of a long-time diabetic, and was extremely reluctant to allow any change in his diet. He claimed to know everything about his own diabetic condition, but surprisingly never even checked his blood sugar levels pre- or post-meal. Instead, he would ask his cook what was prepared for lunch or dinner and adjust his insulin dosage accordingly. When I explained to him that his method was extremely dangerous and would put him at risk for either hypoglycemia or hyperglycemia, he merely shrugged his shoulders and said that the onus of that would be on the cook, for either cooking an insipid meal or a very tasty one! If, for example, the baingan bharta did not taste good he would not eat too much, but since he had already injected himself with a certain amount of insulin, his blood sugar levels would dip within an hour of eating his meal. However, if the cook had prepared a scrumptious baingan bharta, Devendra would overeat and his blood sugar level would rise rapidly.

In my first session with Devendra, his entire family sat in with him and, much to his chagrin, informed me about his eating habits. Maybe because he was browbeaten into it, or maybe because he actually wanted to, Devendra agreed to take the spice mix prescribed for him (which included flax, dried basil, methi, jeera, dried parsley, white sesame seeds, cinnamon powder, gudmar, fennel seeds, and onion seeds). Since I was already treating members of his immediate family, the prescription was quickly given to the cook who promptly made the spice mix according to my specifications. I also gave him a diet plan which he regulated according to what was cooked at home. As it happened, the family soon went on a holiday to New York where, being a man with an incorrigible sweet tooth, Devendra indulged in cheesecake, tiramisu, and pie. I had already informed him that he could occasionally give in to his cravings as long as it did not become a habit. He had promised to slightly increase his dosage of the prescribed spice mix whenever he ate dessert. Once back, he was happy to report that he had been good and had only eaten five small servings of dessert during the entire three-week trip!

Two months later, his endocrinologist had reduced his insulin dosage by six units and had promised to further reduce the insulin dosage if Devendra continued to show a decrease in his blood sugar levels for the next six months. Three months later, he showed me the reduced readings and, grinning sheepishly, he shook hands with me and said that maybe he did not know everything about diabetes after all!

Noninsulin-dependent Diabetes Mellitus (NIDDM)

The much more common form of primary diabetes mellitus (NIDDM) is also known as Type 2 DM or adult onset DM. It usually has an insidious onset. Since the mild symptoms include very minimal to moderate increases in the patients' blood sugar levels, the condition may go undetected for weeks, months, or even years. It is only when the patient seeks medical attention for one of the complications of the disease that the doctor may ask for blood sugar tests and thereby diagnose NIDDM.

Noninsulin-dependent diabetes mellitus (NIDDM) does not result in diabetes ketoacidosis (DKA) if it is left untreated. The NIDDM patient does not need exogenous insulin if he is able to follow a strict diet and exercise regimen. Very often, an oral hypoglycemic agent is sufficient to keep the blood sugars as near to the normal values as possible. Many people with NIDDM are insulin users because they are unable to consistently follow a diet and exercise pattern. They use exogenous insulin because it helps them feel better and achieve better sugar readings rather than because their life solely depends on it.

In NIDDM, insulin deficiency may be described as relative rather than absolute. In some cases the amount of insulin secreted by the pancreas is more than normal, but the condition of insulin resistance is present. If the patient has insulin resistance then the beta cells of the islets of Langerhans produce sufficient amounts of the hormone insulin but the body cells become resistant to this hormone and do not use it effectively to convert sugar into energy, leading thereby to an increase in the blood sugar levels (hyperglycemia). In other cases of Type 2 diabetes, the functioning of the pancreas is altered so that its ability to produce and secrete insulin is reduced. This again leads to elevated blood sugar levels (hyperglycemia).

Diet and exercise play a key role in the successful management of NIDDM and the restoration of the blood sugar levels to values as near to the normal ones as possible. This mainly holds true for a very large percentage of the population with Type 2 diabetes who are above ideal body weight at the time of diagnosis. A diabetic educator along with a nutritionist and a fitness trainer can help an NIDDM patient achieve this. The basic reduction of the NIDDM patients' calorific intake helps in the control of blood sugar levels. Once the daily calorific intake is decreased then the need for insulin also decreases and a balance between supply and demand is achieved. A major reduction in the daily calorific intake may alter the condition of insulin resistance. In this way, the amount of endogenous insulin produced by the body will be more effective in controlling the blood sugar. Most importantly the loss of weight, however small it may be, will increase the relative amount of insulin produced in relation to body weight. As a result of this increased amount of exogenous insulin production, better blood sugar control is achieved. Morbidly overweight patients and sometimes even marginally overweight NIDDM patients may be advised exogenous insulin initially. This is done so that they can achieve better control of their blood sugars in a shorter period of time and in the process lose some weight too. The NIDDM patient who is put on exogenous insulin needs to know that this course of treatment is not lifelong. If this course of treatment is initiated early in the diagnosis of the disease and there is better blood sugar control then the patient may eventually need to get off the exogenous insulin and use oral hypoglycemic, and diet and exercise therapy to maintain near to normal blood sugar values.

NIDDM patients who are at normal weight at the time of diagnosis of the disease often require only an alteration in their basic diet and an increase in their physical activity in order to control their blood sugar. However, sometimes if they are stressed, they benefit from small doses of exogenous insulin in addition to a diet and exercise regimen. Since the normal-weight NIDDM patients retain some of the activity of the beta cells of the pancreas, it is fairly easy to stabilize their blood sugar levels and keep them as near as normal.

Ajinkya Majumdar, a 48-year-old stockbroker, had been diagnosed with NIDDM twelve years previously. Due to constant fluctuations in the stock market his work stress was very high. This, coupled with sleep apnoea and high blood pressure, made it difficult for Ajinkya to keep his blood sugar levels under control. His busy schedule and erratic lifestyle gave him no time to exercise. His dietary pattern was also not a healthy one. Ajinkya's wife Niharika barely got any sleep due to his loud snoring, and was irritated most of the time.

When I first met Ajinkya, his BP was 164/89, FBS was 189, PPBS was 264, and HbA1C was 8.9. These high levels were a cause for concern and his wife was glad that these elevated levels had finally shocked him into seeking help. I first prescribed a detox spice mix which included flax, dried mint, dried celery, cinnamon, jeera, and green elaichi. He was put on a 1600-calorie diabetic diet and was asked to walk for thirty-five minutes four days a week. Within three weeks, his FBS had come down to 145 and PPBS to 203. Subsequently, I also prescribed gudmar and fenugreek seeds in his spice mix.

The next time I met him, his BP had reduced to 137/81 and his FBS to 128, but surprisingly his PPBS still remained at 200. In an attempt to find out what was going on, I asked him to list all the food he ate through the day. As it turned out, Niharika had stopped packing mithai in his lunch dabba, and Ajinkya had taken to eating a lump of jaggery immediately after lunch! I advised him to eat a date the next time he had a sugar craving and, within a week's time, his PPBS came down to 183.

After three months, he reported that his BP was 132/79, FBS was 99, PPBS was 153, and HbA1C was 7.1. Niharika called to say that she was sleeping soundly for the first time in years, since her husband's snoring had become minimal.

All DM patients should be encouraged to monitor their blood sugar levels regularly, even if they feel fine. This is because careful monitoring will reveal any elevations quickly and will enable the healthcare professional to make the necessary adjustments in insulin, drugs, diet, and exercise in order to ensure better management of the disease.

Diseases of the Exocrine Pancreas

If for any reason there is injury to the pancreas, diabetes can result. This can be due to extensive infection of the pancreas which leads to a decrease in the functioning of the pancreatic gland, pancreatitis or inflammation of the pancreas, the surgical removal of the pancreas (pancreatectomy), and even neoplasia and cancer of the pancreatic gland. Sometimes cystic fibrosis damages the beta cells of the islets of Langerhans in the pancreas thereby preventing the proper secretion of the hormone insulin.

Drug-induced Diabetes

There are many drugs which can block the proper secretion of insulin. This decrease in insulin production can result in diabetes. Although these drugs themselves do not cause diabetes, people with insulin resistance using these drugs can be predisposed towards developing the disease. In some rare cases, the beta cells of the pancreas can get totally destroyed because of these drugs. Nicotinic acid and glucocorticosteroids can hamper the proper action of insulin. Other drugs include Vacor, thyroid hormones, Thiazides, Diazoxide, Dilantin, and alpha interferon. Recently statins, a class of medication prescribed by cardiologists to treat high LDL (low-density lipoprotein) cholesterol levels, have been found to modestly increase the risk of developing diabetes mellitus. Steroids, some diuretics, and a few anti-depressants can affect a patient's blood glucose levels.

Genetic Syndromes that are associated with Diabetes

An increase in the incidence of diabetes can sometimes be the result of a genetic syndrome. These include the chromosomal abnormalities of:
- Down's syndrome (or trisomy 21, which is the most common chromosomal abnormality in human beings)
- Klinefelter's syndrome (caused by an additional X chromosome in males, it results in hypogonadism and sterility)
- Turner's syndrome (also known as gonadal dysgenesis in females and characterized by short stature, edema, webbed necks, broad chest, malfunctioning ovaries, and no menstrual cycle leading to sterility)

- Wolfram's syndrome (an autosomal recessive disorder characterized by insulin-deficient diabetes, the absence of β-cells of the islets of Langerhans of the pancreas, optic atrophy, neural deafness, and also hypogonadism)
- Huntington's chorea (a neurodegenerative genetic disease which results in impaired glucose tolerance)

Gestational Diabetes Mellitus (GDM)

As the name suggests, this type of diabetes occurs during pregnancy. When a pregnant female who has never been previously diagnosed as having elevated blood sugars, shows hyperglycemia during any stage of her pregnancy, she is classified as gestational diabetic. In most cases of gestational diabetes, the diagnosis is in the third trimester of the pregnancy. Some women have very high levels of glucose in their blood and their bodies are unable to produce enough insulin to transport all of the glucose into their cells, resulting in progressively rising blood glucose levels.

Women with polycystic ovarian disease are at a greater risk of developing gestational diabetes, as are women with a family history of diabetes, obesity and also women who conceive at an older age (generally above the age of thirty-five). Gestational diabetic women can very often control their blood sugar levels with simple dietary modifications and also with exercise. However 10–20 per cent of women diagnosed with gestational diabetes will have to take some kind of blood glucose-controlling medication.

Children born to women with gestational diabetes are most often larger in size because of the increase in sugar levels of the amniotic fluid. This could lead to complications during their delivery and also caesarean sections. The largest baby I have seen born to a gestational diabetic woman was nearly 12 pounds (5.45 kg) and he looked like a three-month old baby an hour after his birth!

The blood sugar levels generally come back to normal once the baby is born but women diagnosed with gestational diabetes should continue to be careful about their diets because they are at a risk of developing diabetes during later pregnancies or even later on in life. Children, born to gestational diabetic or regular diabetic mothers, may experience a sudden dip in their blood glucose level immediately after birth. They also run the risk of developing diabetes later on in life.

Tara, an aspiring actor and playwright, and Nelson Gill, her banker husband, had been married for eleven years when Tara conceived for the first time. She was very anxious about the growth of the foetus and each time she went for an ultrasonogram, she went prepared to hear bad news. This was primarily because Tara had been diagnosed with gestational diabetes and also with hypothyroidism in her eighteenth week of pregnancy. She had also developed oedema.

When I first met her in her fifth month of pregnancy, Tara had already visited an endocrinologist who prescribed medication for diabetes and hypothyroidism which she was taking diligently. Her doctors had warned her against gaining more than 9 kg totally throughout her gestation period but unfortunately she had put on 57 kg in the first five months itself.

Tara's condition was deteriorating rapidly. Her BP was fairly high partly due to her high stress levels. Her FBS was 76 but her PPBS was 289. Her thyroid-stimulating hormone (TSH) levels were at 11.7. The oedema around her ankles made walking very painful. The water retention significantly contributed to her weight gain.

Her spice-mix prescription (which included flax, cinnamon, dried curry leaves, jeera, saunf, and fenugreek seeds) did not include gudmar because of her thyroid condition. I also advised her to put two stalks of celery in two litres of water and to drink it daily from morning till 7 pm. This would help regulate her blood pressure and bring down her water retention. Within a week of starting the spice mix, Tara reported a decrease in her oedematous condition. After three weeks she repeated her blood tests. Her PPBS level was down to 212 and her TSH reading had reduced to 9. Her relief was palpable and she was extremely happy. She was eating healthy foods and had no craving for savoury snacks, especially those midnight binges during which time she previously used to devour bags of wafers and bowls of deep-fried namkeen. Most importantly, she had not gained any weight in that three-week period.

A month later, Tara gained a meager 650 gm, her FBS was 79, PPBS was 147, and TSH level was down to 7.3. I asked her to add kasoori methi and coriander to her spice mix. Since her blood pressure had stabilized and water retention had gone, she no longer needed celery in her therapeutic water. I now advised her to add half a teaspoon of roasted ajwain to two litres of her therapeutic water to help her with digestion.

By the time she was due for delivery, she had gained a total of 12.2 kg, her FBS was 72, PPBS was 130, and TSH level had decreased to 5.5. Baby Urvi was born at thirty-nine weeks of gestation and weighed a healthy 9 pounds. Her parents dote on her and she is the light of their lives. Tara and her husband were very happy with the way in which her first pregnancy progressed after her fifth month of gestation. Since Urvi is now four, they are extremely keen on planning for their second child. This time Tara promises to seek my help even before she conceives!

2

The Complications of Diabetes

Diabetes is a condition in which glucose circulating in the bloodstream cannot be absorbed properly. Since blood travels throughout the body, whenever there is too much glucose present in it, the viscosity of the blood changes. This, in turn, causes disruptions in the normal chemical environment that the organ systems of the body function within. Hence the body starts to show signs that things are not working properly inside. This manifests in the complications of diabetes. If diabetes is left untreated and major fluctuations in blood glucose levels are not addressed immediately, it can lead to a number of serious complications. When dramatic rise and fall in blood glucose levels is a common occurrence, there can be serious consequences in terms of health. This can leave a diabetic patient susceptible to heart attacks, strokes, diabetic retinopathy or eye damage and glaucoma, diabetic nephropathy or kidney damage, vascular disease or blood vessel disease that may require an amputation, tooth and gum or periodontal disease, skin and mucous membrane infections, respiratory tract infections, urinary tract infections, diabetic neuropathy or nerve damage, and impotence in men. Diabetic coma can be fatal. Type 1 diabetic women should be very careful about maintaining their blood glucose level to as near as normal because they can develop menstrual irregularities, polycystic ovarian syndrome, infertility, and even early menopause.

The disturbing list of symptoms, coupled with the fact that a complete cure for diabetes has yet to be found, may sound like a life sentence. I feel sad when a newly diagnosed diabetic asks if he has to follow the diet restrictions for the rest of his life. I have no answers for the parent of a diabetic infant who ask the same question. I once met a mother whose two-year-old had been diagnosed with diabetes and what she had to say was heart-wrenching: she would monitor his diet, insulin injections, etc. day and night but would say a prayer and leave him in the hands of God each time she dropped him off to playschool, because she was never sure about how much of gooey chocolate cake he would manage to get his little hands on each time his classmates celebrated their birthday in school. She and her husband would take turns to check on him at two-hourly intervals through the night just to ensure that his blood glucose levels had not dipped.

The good news is that prevention plays an important role in keeping these complications at bay. By maintaining a tight control of his blood glucose, a diabetic patient can help his body function as normally as possible. Tight control on blood glucose can help decrease the chances of complications occurring from elevated glucose levels. Other health problems can accelerate the harmful effect of diabetes. These include high blood cholesterol levels, high blood pressure, thyroid malfunction, obesity, stress, alcohol and drug abuse, smoking, and the lack of regular physical exercise. Diabetics need regular monitoring in order to maintain their blood glucose levels, liver profile, renal profile, blood pressure, and cholesterol levels as near to normal as possible. These will go a long way in delaying or preventing the onset of the various complications associated with this disorder. The most important thing is to maintain a positive frame of mind and be confident that you can overcome the complications associated with this metabolic disorder. Family help, support, and encouragement will go a long way in achieving this. Extreme weight loss with the help of a gastric bypass surgery can reverse some cases of Type 2 diabetes.

Hyperglycemia

Hyperglycemia occurs when the blood glucose levels rise much above the normal values (generally above 200 mg/dl). A number of complications arise because of this but the scary part is that symptoms of hyperglycemia are often unnoticed even when the blood glucose level crosses 300 mg/dl. There are many reasons why the blood glucose levels can reach these high values. Uncontrolled diabetes, failure to take diabetic medication on time, eating large amounts of carbohydrate-rich food, lack of exercise, infections, critical illness, physical and mental stress, pregnancy, menstruation, and the intake of certain drugs like antipsychotic medications can all contribute towards a spike in the blood glucose level.

Diabetic Ketoacidosis (DKA)

Hyperglycemia is a serious problem and it should be treated as soon as it is detected. Failure to do so can lead to a condition called Diabetic Ketoacidosis (DKA), which is always a medical emergency for which the diabetic patient has to be hospitalized. When a diabetic patient develops DKA, there is an acute elevation in the blood sugar level (400–800 mg/dl and sometimes even more). It occurs when the body has insufficient amounts of the hormone insulin. This low insulin causes the liver to turn fatty acid for fuel. The body needs glucose for energy, but when insulin is not present in sufficient amounts, the cells cannot have access to the high levels of glucose circulating in the blood and so fats are broken down to be used for energy. This in turn leads to a surge in the amount of waste products called ketone bodies being produced which increase the pH of the blood. These ketones have to be removed through the urine.

If this process of removal of ketone bodies does not happen on time then they accumulate in the bloodstream leading to ketoacidosis or diabetic coma. A patient with DKA is admitted into hospital with shortness of breath or deep breathing, fruity or acetone-smelling breath, and dry or parched mouth that is often accompanied by abdominal pain, dehydration, nausea, and vomiting. If not treated on time, DKA can lead to coma and death. Hence all diabetic patients should have an identification tag that simply reads 'DIABETIC'. In an emergency, this will help bystanders identify that the person who has lost consciousness at an airport, railway station, etc. is a diabetic and not leave him lying there assuming he is alcohol intoxicated, like what recently happened at Mumbai Airport. IDDM patients are more prone to DKA than NIDDM patients. Insulin administration is crucial in the quick management of DKA.

Whenever a patient's blood glucose levels are high I advise them to decrease their carbohydrate intake, and start consuming a spice mix that includes flax, fenugreek (both in dried leaf as well as seed form), *Gymnema sylvestre* leaves or gudmar (if they do not have a malfunctioning thyroid gland) chia seeds, coriander seeds, cumin and cinnamon, immediately after meals and to increase or intensify their exercise schedule. Exercise can help in bringing the blood glucose levels down. If, however, the blood glucose levels cross 220 mg/dl, I ask them to check if there are ketone bodies in the urine via a urine test. Patients with ketones in their urine are asked to refrain from exercising as exercise can make the level of glucose in the blood stream climb even higher. The best way to work on this is to quickly consult your diabetologist or healthcare practitioner.

Hypoglycemia

Hypoglycemia occurs when the insulin supply is so high that practically all the glucose moves out of the bloodstream and goes into the cells. Due to this, the brain gets starved of fuel and the patient can go into coma. Hypoglycemia usually presents itself as abnormally low levels of blood glucose causing agitation, cold sweats, convulsions, and the inability to think clearly which may cause a panic attack, loss of consciousness leading to coma, and seizures; if left untreated, hypoglycemia can lead to brain damage and death. Hypoglycemia may be caused if the diabetic patient has been administered too much insulin or has eaten too little carbohydrates in a particular meal or both. Since exercise decreases a diabetic patient's insulin requirements, too much exercise can also lead to hypoglycemia; this is especially true if the patient takes his regular recommended dosage of insulin despite having completed a strenuous bout of exercise.

The most common way to treat hypoglycemia is to give

the patient a glass of fruit juice or a sweetened beverage like nimbu pani or even a date or a piece of chocolate or toffee. Care should be taken to ensure judicious usage of these sugary drinks or snacks else the patient will go into hyperglycemia. In severe cases, when the patient is unconscious and has been admitted to hospital, a glucagon injection is given to stabilize the blood glucose level.

Glucagon, produced by the alpha cells of the islets of Langerhans of the pancreas, raises blood sugar levels and thus its effect is the exact opposite of the hormone insulin which lowers the blood sugar levels. At other times, the unconscious hypoglycemic patient is administered dextrose through an intravenous drip. Most hospitals prefer to use the dextrose drip.

Periodontal Disease

When blood glucose levels are not properly managed, it can lead to gum disease. Periodontitis is a lesser known complication of diabetes. Periodontal disease can affect the gums of a diabetic patient, as well as the bone which holds the teeth in place. If the blood sugar is not under control then saliva can contain higher than normal levels of glucose which in turn encourages the growth of disease-producing bacteria, especially in the gums. Patients with periodontitis often complain of halitosis or bad breath, receding gums, loosening of the teeth, and gum bleeds whilst they are brushing their teeth or flossing or even biting into fruit. Dentists observe the presence of pus in the gums or between the teeth; swollen, tender, red gums (a classic characteristic of gingivitis); and sometimes even changes in the jaw alignment. This is because high blood glucose levels can affect and weaken the gums and bones. Regular chewing on stalks of celery can help prevent halitosis. A tulsi–haldi (basil–turmeric) gargle will prevent pus formation. Massaging of the gums with salt will help strengthen them but please ensure that you gargle well to rinse off the salt, especially if you have high blood pressure.

Respiratory Tract Infections

The immune system of a diabetic patient is greatly compromised if he does not maintain a tight control of his blood glucose level. Each time the blood glucose level increases, the cells get inflamed and this causes a reduction in immune cell function. Diabetes is a known risk factor in the development of lower respiratory tract infections and diabetics with poor blood glucose control are most susceptible to pulmonary or lung infections, tuberculosis, pneumonia, and influenza. Unfortunately, when there is poor control over blood glucose, these respiratory infections are of greater intensity and show a slower period of recovery. Also, because of the infection, the blood glucose level rises which further hampers the recovery process.

The immune system can be strengthened by introducing glutathione to the diet. This nutrient helps the immune system fight infections. It is a powerful antioxidant and is most plentiful in the red, pulpy area of the watermelon near the rind. I recommend it even though watermelons have a high glycemic index. Glutathione can also be found in broccoli, Brussels sprouts, cabbage, cauliflower, spinach, and other cruciferous vegetables.

A good remedy to treat a cold as well as a dry cough that a diabetic patient can try is to make a brew of 2 tablespoons of ginger juice, 1 tablespoon of garlic juice, a pinch of haldi powder, a pinch of cinnamon powder, 10 fenugreek seeds, and 2 green elaichi in 100 ml water. Bring to a boil and allow it to simmer for two minutes. Strain it, add 1 teaspoon of lime juice, and drink while it is warm. Repeat this two to three times a day until the cough and cold subsides. Alternatively, put the above mentioned ingredients into a thermos filled with 1 litre of hot water and drink this water through the day.

URINARY TRACT INFECTIONS

Bacteria in the urine (bacteriuria), cystitis, fungal infections leading to infections in the urinary tract are a common occurrence in women with diabetes, who show poor blood glucose control. The high concentration of sugar in the urine further aggravates this problem and increases the time taken for the infection to heal. This can lead to poor bladder control and urinary incontinence in both diabetic males as well as diabetic females. Unsweetened cranberry juice and cranberry tablets help to a great extent, as do botanical diuretic herbs like dandelion, celery, parsley, and stinging nettle. Teas made from these herbs are readily available at health food stores. It goes without saying that once the blood glucose levels are better controlled, the patient will find faster relief from urinary tract infections. If the infection is severe, it is best to consult your healthcare practitioner at the earliest.

For mild urinary tract infections and burning micturation drink 2 litres of water infused with 2 stalks of celery, 10 mint leaves, 1 tablespoon of dried coriander seeds, and the juice of 1 lemon. It is best to drink this water between 9 am and 7 pm.

Skin Problems

Diabetes affects almost all parts of the body, including the skin. This is because blood reaches all the different parts of the body. At least 35 per cent of all diabetics experience some or the other type of skin problem in their lifetime. Some skin issues such as acanthosis nigricans can be a warning sign of impaired glucose tolerance and insulin resistance. The skin around the nape of the neck, elbows, and knees creases and armpit skin darkens and becomes thick. Blood glucose levels should be checked regularly. Type 1 diabetics are more prone to vitiligo than Type 2 diabetics. Vitiligo affects the colour of the skin. Cells that make the skin pigment melanin, which gives the skin its colour, are destroyed, leaving patches of discoloured skin especially on the chest and back. Infected foot ulcers can develop if there is neuropathy. A blister caused by an ill-fitting shoe can develop into an open sore or ulcer. Bacterial infections like styes on the eyelids, boils, nail infections, and carbuncles make the area around the infection very painful. Fungal infections like candida albicans, athlete's foot, jock itch, vaginal infections, and ringworm can cause itchy red rashes and blisters. Poor circulation and yeast infections can cause dry, itchy skin, mainly on the lower legs. When there is poor blood glucose control, high blood cholesterol, and triglyceride levels, eruptive xanthomatosis can occur. Red-ringed, firm, yellow, pea-sized bumps which can itch a lot, develop on the backs of the hands, arms, feet, and sometimes on the buttocks. As with all other problems associated with diabetes, maintaining a tight control on the blood glucose values can help prevent, decrease the intensity, or even cure these skin problems.

Angiopathy

Chronic elevation of blood glucose level leads to the damage of blood vessels. This is known as angiopathy. When the small blood vessels are damaged it is known as microangiopathy. When the arteries are damaged it is known as macroangiopathy.

Microangiopathy can lead to:
- Diabetic cardiomyopathy, which is a malfunctioning of the ventricles of the heart irrespective of coronary artery disease and high blood pressure. It damages the heart, causes diastolic and systolic dysfunction, and leads to heart failure. It is essential to control blood glucose levels, keep blood pressure as close to normal as possible, and treat ischaemic heart disease in order to prevent as also to treat diabetic cardiomyopathy.
- Diabetic retinopathy, which occurs when there is swelling of the macula and the growth of poor-quality blood vessels which supply blood to the retina. The eyes are filled with tiny blood vessels called capillaries. Excess blood glucose can damage these capillaries. Diabetic retinopathy is common in patients who have diabetes for a long time (20 or more years), are insulin users, have high levels of HbA1c (generally above 9), high blood cholesterol, and higher systolic blood pressure. If diabetic retinopathy is not treated on time it can lead to severe loss of vision or total blindness. All diabetics should be encouraged to have regular eye examinations, especially of the retina, and to keep their blood glucose, blood cholesterol, and blood pressure under control.
- Diabetic nephropathy, which affects the kidneys. Like the

eyes, the kidneys are also filled with tiny blood vessels or capillaries which can get damaged when there is a chronic increase in the blood glucose levels. Very often, diabetic nephropathy can lead to total malfunction of the kidneys. Reducing blood glucose levels can minimize this damage. Diabetic nephropathy can be reversed or controlled with a good renal diabetic diet in which protein restriction is sometimes needed, as is the prevention of electrolyte depletion. If good care is not taken then the patient will need renal dialysis.

- Diabetic neuropathy occurs when the nerve ends get damaged as a result of large amounts of glucose passing through the small blood vessels or capillaries. This can be even more damaging when the blood pressure is also very high. Diabetic neuropathy initially affects the hands and feet. A patient with uncontrolled diabetes and neuropathy will experience a typical burning, tingling, and pins-and-needles feeling in the hands and feet, called peripheral neuropathy. Over a period of time this can progress to total loss of sensation or numbness, especially in the feet. Once the patient's feet lose sensation then his balance gets affected and he is not able to walk properly. This is scary because the patient is unable to notice injuries and burns. Diabetic neuropathy can impair proper blood circulation and cause diabetic foot. Hence diabetics should get their feet checked regularly and take utmost care while clipping their toe nails. Patients with diabetic foot are more susceptible to skin ulcers of the feet. If not treated on time, it can lead to delay in the healing of infected wounds and more scarily to necrosis or the death of the cells of the skin, gangrene, and amputation of the toes and the feet.

Diabetic neuropathy can also lead to digestive problems and erectile dysfunction.
- ➢ Diabetic encephalopathy, which occurs when there are changes in the central nervous system. Uncontrolled diabetes can cause neuropsychiatric complications, cognitive decline, depression, anxiety, and dementia. There is damage to the neurons of the brain due to high levels of blood glucose. Diabetics are advised to take curcumin or haldi which is a well-known antioxidant and anti-inflammatory agent which protects the neurons of the brain from damage.

Macroangiopathy can lead to cardiovascular disease. Atherosclerosis contributes to this:
- ➢ Coronary heart disease. When a diabetic patient has poor control over his ailment, his triglycerides (blood fats) are usually elevated. This puts him at a greater risk of developing coronary heart disease. The arteries that supply blood to the heart, to enable the heart to function properly, now clog up and prevent sufficient amounts of blood from reaching the heart. This impairs heart function. A diabetic should regularly test his blood lipid levels. It is best to maintain a low level of fasting serum triglyceride (less than 150 mg/dl) and a high level of the good cholesterol faction, i.e., HDL (high-dencity lipoprotein) cholesterol (more than 40 mg/dl). This is because a rise in the ratio of serum triglyceride to HDL cholesterol (more than 3.5) is a predictor of coronary heart disease. Flaxseed, chia seeds, melon seeds, sunflower seeds, walnuts, and pumpkin seeds should be included in a low-fat diet to keep the heart healthy. Regular exercise is also essential because it increases

the rate at which blood glucose is used up. Coronary heart disease can lead to angina or pain in the heart muscle and myocardial infarction or heart attack and stroke.

3

Myths and FAQs

Ever since my first internship at KEM Hospital, Mumbai in 1990 and subsequently at the S.L. Raheja Hospital, Mumbai which at that time exclusively dealt with diabetes, I have been working with diabetic patients to help them achieve optimum blood glucose levels without increasing oral hypoglycemic medications and insulin dosage. Since the disease is so widespread, everybody knows somebody who has diabetes. When someone is diagnosed with the ailment, there are many friends and relatives who offer advice, most of it being non-scientific. The diagnosis of the metabolic disease can be hard on the patient as well as his family members as they struggle to cope with a number of changes in their daily life, the most important of these being the daily food menu. Parents of diabetic children often ask when their child will outgrow the disease. Most people believe that eating something bitter like karela or methi will never allow for their blood sugar levels to rise, especially after eating mithai. This shows that there is a lack of knowledge about the disease.

I often meet diabetics with uncontrolled blood glucose levels who are not very concerned about their ailment. This is because there are many myths about diabetes that make it difficult for people to believe that it is a serious and potentially fatal disease. They do not realize that their lax attitude towards the ailment can have serious and life-threatening implications. Most of the time these patients have relatives with the same disease and feel that if their parent/sibling does not have any complications related to uncontrolled diabetes, they too will not experience any complications. When it comes to living and coping with diabetes, what the diabetic patient thinks he knows about the disease from relatives and friends can be worse than what he does not know. This is because non-scientific information and uninformed thinking can come in the way of good medical care and better blood glucose control. Here are some of the common myths and fallacies related to the disease along with explanations to demystify the same:

Myth 1: Eating refined sugar causes diabetes.

So widespread is this myth that refined sugar is now banned from many homes and people without this metabolic disease have switched to even more harmful sugar substitutes like aspartame. Type 2 diabetes may be caused by the inability of the pancreas to produce sufficient amounts of the hormone insulin, or due to insulin resistance. Being overweight can contribute to impaired glucose metabolism. Overeating all types of carbohydrates and fats and not exercising sufficiently can cause weight gain. Drinking sugary drinks on a daily basis can put one at risk for developing diabetes. A 12 oz can of sweetened aerated beverage or sports/energy drink or fruit juice provides carbohydrate equivalent to ten teaspoons of sugar! Hence one should limit the intake of these beverages.

Myth 2: Only older people get diabetes.

More than 20 years ago, when I started consulting at a diabetes clinic in Mumbai, if a child or an adolescent was diagnosed with diabetes it was always Type 1. This is not the case anymore. Sadly, today children as young as eight and ten years of age are being diagnosed with Type 2 diabetes. I use the word 'sadly' because the onset of Type 2 diabetes is associated with an unhealthy diet and lifestyle. The onus of inculcating good habits lies with the parents. Children should be encouraged to eat more wholesome food and less junk food, spend more time on the football field or in the swimming pool and less time in front of the television or computer, and should not be immensely pressurized to perform as well as or better than their peers.

To help prevent diabetes in children, parents should try to encourage good habits for the entire family. That means less video game and TV time, more physical activity, less junk food, and smaller portions.

Myth 3: Diabetes being a common ailment, it is not a serious disease.

Sadly, the fact of the matter is that diabetes causes more deaths than AIDS and breast cancer combined. Type 2 diabetics may have the disease for many years before it is diagnosed, because they feel that the symptoms will go away and therefore do not test their blood glucose levels. They may even make excuses for the symptoms rather than visit the doctor and get the required tests done. For example, they will attribute extreme thirst to the weather, excessive urination at night to drinking more water in the latter half of the day, blurry vision to computer-associated eye stress, etc. An early diagnosis can help ward off many of the life-threatening complications associated with the disease. Diabetes can be controlled with effort and care. As long as you regularly test your blood glucose level and take steps to maintain the level as near to normal as possible, complications associated with the disease will not arise. A diabetic patient is susceptible to heart attacks, retinopathy, nephropathy, neuropathy, encephalopathy, periodontal disease, respiratory tract infections, urinary tract infections, and skin infections.

MYTH 4: TYPE 2 DIABETES IS NOT AS SERIOUS AS TYPE 1.

Type 1 and type 2 diabetes are equally serious, because when poorly controlled they both can lead to the same devastating and life-threatening complications like heart attack; stroke; eye damage and blindness; kidney damage and kidney failure; nerve damage; toe, foot, and leg amputation; brain damage; gum disease; lung disease and respiratory tract infections; UTIs (urinary tract infections); and sexual dysfunction.

MYTH 5: DIABETIC WOMEN SHOULD NOT GET PREGNANT.

Due to the widespread availability of self blood-glucose monitoring kits and other technologies that allow the mother-to-be to fine-tune her blood glucose levels as close to the normal levels as possible, diabetic women with either Type 1 or Type 2 diabetes can get pregnant, carry full term without any complications, and deliver normal and healthy babies.

At least six months before she is planning to conceive, a diabetic woman should consult her diabetologist, gynaecologist, and nutritionist and work with them to maintain a tight control on her blood glucose levels as well as her blood pressure and blood cholesterol levels. This control should continue to be maintained throughout the nine-month gestation period and would then allow for a healthy diabetic pregnancy and a complication-free normal delivery of a healthy baby.

Myth 6: Diabetes is an infectious disease.

'My husband has diabetes. Will I get it too?' 'My child's classmate has been diagnosed with IDDM. Should I ask my son to stop playing with him so that he too will not get diabetes?' These are questions I am sometimes asked, which indicate how little people know about the disease even though its prevalence is widespread. Diabetes is not contagious. It cannot be caught like the flu, conjunctivitis, or an STD (sexually transmitted disease). Genetics and lifestyle make one susceptible to the disease as does a disease of the pancreas.

Myth 7: All overweight and obese people will develop diabetes.

One of the many risk factors for developing diabetes is being overweight. However, not all overweight people with a Body Mass Index (BMI) over 25 will develop diabetes. In fact, many NIDDM patients are of normal weight or are very slightly overweight at the time of diagnosis. Some are even underweight, raising the possibility that undernourishment can be a possible risk factor. However, being obese, i.e., having a BMI of 30 or more, is considered to be a major risk factor for developing diabetes.

Myth 8 : Diabetics are prone to coughs, colds, and other illnesses.

As long as a diabetic keeps a tight control on his blood glucose level, he can lead a healthy life. He is as susceptible to a common cold and other infection as a non-diabetic. However, any other illness can make diabetes more difficult to control. In fact, some medications commonly prescribed for infections can increase the blood glucose levels for the duration that they are being consumed. Hence diabetics are often advised to take precautionary measures whenever there is an epidemic. Consuming foods rich in antioxidants like fresh fruit and vegetables, green tea, etc. can increase immunity.

Myth 9: Insulin cures diabetes.

Unfortunately, till date, no complete cure has been found for diabetes. Research in this field is still on. Insulin is necessary for IDDM. Bariatric surgery can help obese individuals bring their weight down and reverse NIDDM. Insulin injections help both IDDM and NIDDM patients keep the blood glucose under control.

Myth 10: If the diabetologist puts the NIDDM patient on insulin, it means the patient has been lax and that it is the beginning of the end.

When a person has been diagnosed with NIDDM and his

blood glucose levels are slightly above normal, it is possible to bring these levels to normal with diet and exercise. Since diabetes is a progressive disease, oral hypoglycemic medications may be needed along with diet and exercise. Over time, the pancreas gets more sluggish and produces lesser and lesser amounts of its own insulin. At this point, rather than increasing the dosage of oral hypoglycemic medications, diabetologists recommend insulin injections for better control of the disease. This may sometimes be for a short period of time, depending on the patient's glucose response. Once on insulin, the diabetic should be encouraged to regularly monitor his glucose levels and any signs of hypoglycemia should be immediately reported to the doctor.

Many people are dismayed when their diabetologist finally puts them on insulin. You cannot really blame them. For years their doctor has threatened to put them on insulin if they do not show improved results. They feel they have failed. They associate going on insulin injections with worsening diabetes, or they believe that insulin causes complications. Far from being 'the beginning of the end', for most people, starting insulin is the 'beginning of better health'. They have better blood glucose control, which in turn gives them more energy and less fatigue, clearer vision, sleeping through the night, and possibly halting or reversing complications.

People also believe that insulin causes diabetic complications, such as numbness, blindness, kidney failure, and lower-limb amputation. This is possibly because they have seen a relative or friend suffer such consequences shortly after beginning insulin therapy. But in these patients, complications result not from using insulin, but rather from many prior years of uncontrolled blood glucose levels.

Myth 11 : Diabetics should avoid desserts.

A diabetic requires a healthy meal plan which includes all nutrients in amounts necessary to maintain good health. Moderation is key. Limiting desserts will help keep blood glucose under control, but most of the time the patient ends up feeling deprived and frustrated about not being able to enjoy a meal out with friends and family. An occasional indulgence in a small serving of dessert can be incorporated into a meal plan as long as it is preceded and also followed by a bout of exercise to help burn off the extra sugar. During hypoglycemia, a small portion of chocolate/candy can help bring the blood glucose level back into the normal range.

Myth 12: Bread, rice, pasta, and potato are taboo for diabetics.

I meet many diabetics who are perplexed about their rising blood glucose levels despite taking a badha (a religious vow) not to eat the foods mentioned above for six months/a year/ forever! I incorporate multigrain bread, brown rice, whole-wheat pasta, and boiled, not fried, potatoes in a diabetic diet. Here too, moderation is the key.

Myth 13: Fruit has sugar and should be avoided by diabetics.

Fruit is a healthy food containing vitamins, minerals, fibre, antioxidants, and digestive enzymes required for good health. Therefore, fruit should be a part of a healthy meal plan. Fruit also contains fruit sugar known as fructose. Hence fruit should never be eaten immediately after a meal. It is best eaten on an empty stomach on rising, or as a snack between breakfast and lunch or between lunch and dinner. Eating a fruit before a vigorous exercise programme will prevent the blood glucose levels from falling dangerously low and also provide energy to exercise. If the blood glucose levels do not fall in the middle of the night, a diabetic should avoid eating fruit after dinner or as a late night snack. For better blood glucose control, a diabetic should opt for fruits which have a low glycemic index like apple, kiwi, jamun, and grapefruit. Since grapefruit interferes with the action of statins, diabetics on cholesterol-lowering statin medications should avoid eating this fruit. Grapefruit juice also interferes with the action of antihistamines, certain BP (blood pressure) medications, psychiatric drugs, immunosupressants, pain medication, impotence drugs, and AIDS medication.

Myth 14: Skipping breakfast is a good way to control high blood glucose levels.

Eating a wholesome breakfast is highly recommended, even among those diabetics who are trying to lose weight. For those diabetic patients wishing to maintain or lose weight, the total calories for breakfast or any other meal should be controlled to the desired amount. If the diabetic skips breakfast after more than six hours of fasting while he is asleep, the blood glucose level will go down too low, affecting both mental and physical performance. This can lead to hypoglycemia in the middle of a workday or can cause the patient to eat more than he usually would at lunchtime. As a result, post-lunch glucose levels will rise much more than they normally would. Keeping the pancreas healthy so that the level of insulin secreted is optimum, is important to prevent the onset of diabetes and for general well-being. In order to prevent spikes in serum insulin levels it is always better to eat five to six small meals through the day not exceeding the desired limit of total calories for the day.

Myth 15 : Diabetics should wear special shoes.

Good foot health is imperative for a diabetic patient primarily because of the complications associated with diabetic foot. As long as the shoes are comfortable to walk in, and do not put stress on their feet, diabetics can wear any shoe that fits properly. It is always better to shop for shoes in the latter half of the day when the feet are slightly swollen after standing or walking about for a couple of hours. Shoes with comfortable soles and cushioned insoles should be opted for. The new shoes should be easy to walk in, when tried in the store itself. They should neither cramp the toes nor rub the delicate skin of the feet. Never listen to the salesman who says that the shoes need to be 'broken in'.

II

Managing Diabetes

Diabetes is a lifelong, total-body problem. If a diabetic wants to manage his disorder and his overall health, it is best he understands the disease and is aware of its complications. Managing diabetes requires a great deal of tenacity, a positive frame of mind, and lots of support from family and friends. Every diabetic should constantly strive to keep a tight control on his blood glucose level. Diet is the backbone of both IDDM and NIDDM. It should always be the first line of attack in stabilizing elevated blood glucose levels. Careful and regular monitoring of the blood glucose level, a healthy food and exercise regimen, and medication whenever necessary are the basic strategies in the management of diabetes. Generally, medical solutions seem more focused on a reactionary approach to blood sugar management, that is, the dosage of medication is adjusted according to the glucose readings. It is more crucial to address the underlying imbalance of nutrients that finally lead to the manifestation of diabetes as a symptom of a disease. This nutrient imbalance includes mineral deficiencies of zinc, chromium, manganese, and vanadium. Almost all diabetes management programmes focus on hydrating the body well with a minimum of two litres plain water; increasing the intake of wholegrain, fibre-rich food while limiting the intake of simple carbohydrates, including dietary supplements of zinc, manganese, chromium, and vanadium; and, most importantly, asking the patient to sleep more and indulge in stress-busting activities. A diabetic should be made to realize that his body is more sensitive to any kind of change—physical, physiological, environmental, or mental—than that of a non-diabetic. The human body is the best possible monitor of its own condition, so it is very important to listen to it.

4

Controlling Diabetes with Allopathic Medication

Every diabetic dreads getting his blood glucose level tested. He generally procrastinates and will finally get it done only when a family member or nutritionist or doctor goads or threatens or emotionally blackmails him. The report is received with trepidation because it most often indicates that the patient has been lax and there is need for a new and higher dosage of medication. The major goal in treating diabetes is to decrease blood glucose levels without causing hypoglycemia. This can be achieved only with the compliance of the patient. IDDM or Type 1 diabetes is treated with exogenous insulin, regular exercise and a low-glycemic diabetic diet. NIDDM or Type 2 diabetes is initially treated with weight reduction (if the patient is overweight), a low-glycemic diabetic diet, and regular exercise. When these measures fail to bring down high blood glucose levels, oral hypoglycemic medications are used. If, however, oral hypoglycemic medications do not help the diabetic patient, the diabetologist will look towards exogenous insulin as a form of treatment. This line of treatment does not always mean that the diabetic patient has been lax about his diet and exercise regimen. Over time, the pancreas gets more sluggish and produces lesser and lesser amounts of its own insulin. At this point, rather than increasing the dosage of oral hypoglycemic medication, diabetologists recommend insulin injections for better control of the disease. This may sometimes be for a short period of time, depending on the patient's glucose response.

A balanced, nutritious diet low in saturated fat and simple carbohydrates and high in fibre is generally recommended for controlling blood glucose levels. Even a 20 per cent reduction in body weight can increase sensitivity to insulin and help in better diabetes management. Persons whose diabetes has been well controlled may sometimes suddenly become hyperglycemic in response to an increase in either psychological or physiological stress. It is possible to offset a temporary increase in mild psychological stress by an increase in stress-busting cardiovascular exercise, meditation, and yoga. Regular exercise and stress management help achieve diabetes control in a much better way.

ALLOPATHIC MEDICATION FOR NIDDM OR TYPE 2 DIABETES

Generally, when a diabetologist recommends allopathic medications to a Type 2 diabetic, he is hoping to: increase the pancreatic secretion of the hormone insulin; make the blood cells more sensitive to the hormone insulin; help in slow gastric emptying and prevent quick intestinal carbohydrate absorption so that carbohydrates take a longer time to reach the intestine; and decrease liver glucose release which otherwise reflects in high fasting blood glucose levels. The treatment is always tailor-made to suit an individual patient's needs. Since long-term complications arise from poor diabetes control, strict compliance forms the core of diabetes management. Patients should be educated about the risks associated with the disease so that they do not get lax about its management. Lifestyle modification is the key to a healthier life.

Increase the pancreatic secretion of the hormone insulin:

> **Sulfonylureas**: Medication used to treat NIDDM or Type 2 diabetes should increase the amount of insulin secreted by the pancreas. Sulfonylureas are oral hypoglycemic agents which help control blood glucose levels of Type 2 diabetics by stimulating the beta cells of the islets of Langerhans in the pancreas to produce and release more insulin. This can happen only if these beta cells still retain their capacity to do so. Sulfonylureas include glyburides (Diabeta, Glynase, Micronase), glipizides (Bimode SR, Diaglip, Glide), and glimepirides (Daoryl, Amaryl). These drugs can quickly lower blood glucose levels. However, they can cause hypoglycemia. In addition, they are sulphur-containing drugs and should be avoided by patients who are allergic to sulphur. IDDM or Type 1 diabetics should never be recommended sulfonylureas. Sulfonylureas are generally ineffective in controlling blood sugar level during times of increased stress. Many diabetics will happily take their medication but will procrastinate when it comes to making lifestyle changes. Hence it is important for the diabetologist to explain to the patient that these medications are not a

cure for the disease and they cannot be used as a substitute for diet and exercise.

> **Meglitinides**: These medications also act on the beta cells of the islets of Langerhans of the pancreas to promote insulin secretion. They are short acting and their general peak function is achieved in one hour. They include repaglinides (Eurepa, Novonorm, Q-Repa) and nateglinides (Glinate, Natelide, Natiz) and are recommended for up to a maximum of thrice a day just before meals. Since they are short-acting, they are better at lowering post-meal blood glucose levels as compared to fasting blood glucose levels.

Make the blood cells more sensitive to insulin:

> **Thiazolidinediones**: These medications make the blood cells more sensitive to insulin so that they respond better to the insulin secreted by the pancreas. They make the muscle and fat cells more responsive to insulin. These drugs include pioglitazone and rosiglitazone. A couple of years ago, the Indian government banned the manufacture and sale of rosiglitazone because of concerns about a possible increased risk of cardiovascular side effects such as heart attack and stroke. In June 2013, the sale of pioglitazone was also suspended because of concerns of its association with increased bladder cancer risk. More research is anxiously awaited by Indian diabetologists who feel the new data coming out in 2014 will be in favour of this drug. Regardless of controversy, diabetic patients with cardiovascular disease should not be prescribed thiazolidinediones. Liver profile tests should be frequently done by patients on these drugs

and if the readings cross three times the normal value, these drugs should be stopped immediately.

Help in slow gastric emptying and prevent quick intestinal carbohydrate absorption

➢ **Acarboses** (Glucobay, Precose, Prandase) block alpha glucosidase, the enzyme that breaks down starch and complex sugars into glucose. Before being absorbed into the bloodstream, carbohydrates must be broken down by enzymes into glucose molecules which enter the bloodstream and cause a spike in the blood glucose levels. One of the enzymes from the intestine involved in breaking down carbohydrates is called alpha glucosidase. By inhibiting this enzyme, carbohydrates are not broken down as efficiently and glucose absorption is delayed. In this way, starch and complex carbohydrates do not get digested and pass through the stomach and small intestine instead of converting to glucose and entering the blood stream as soon as a meal is eaten. This is a temporary process, and the starch and complex carbohydrates ultimately do get broken down into glucose and finally enter the bloodstream. This process is a slow one and glucose enters the bloodstream in small amounts rather than in one big glucose spike. Acarboses can have gastrointestinal side effects like flatulence, stomachache and diarrhoea.

Decrease the amount of glucose produced by the liver

➢ **Biguanides** or metformin (Glucophage, Glycomet, Cetapin) have the ability to decrease the production of glucose by the liver. Metformin acts by increasing the sensitivity of liver, muscle, fat, and other tissues to the uptake and also the effects of insulin. These actions lower the level of glucose in the blood. Since metformin does not increase the concentration of insulin in the blood it does not cause excessively low blood glucose levels (hypoglycemia), which is the reason why most diabetologists prefer to prescribe it for NIDDM or Type 2 diabetic patients. Metformin suppresses the appetite thereby helping overweight diabetics lose some weight. It should not be used in patients with kidney disease and should be used with caution in those with liver disease.

INSULIN

When a diabetologist prescribes insulin to a Type 2 diabetic, most patients will resist and promise to come back with better blood glucose readings a few weeks or months later. They feel that insulin injections will now add to the burden of managing their blood glucose levels. This is mostly because of the overwhelming fear of having to inject themselves daily. Some patients feel angry at the doctor for not being able to help them and even consult other diabetologists in the hope that, in this way, they will be able to stave off the onset of the insulin injections. They have heard about the side effects of insulin and are afraid. There is also a sense of failure—that they have not been able to control their diet, that they have been lax with their exercise schedule, that things will now spiral downhill … that this is the end of the world.

As a young dietetic intern at S.L. Raheja Hospital, which at that time catered solely to diabetics, one very vivid memory still brings tears to my eyes: a seven-year-old recently diagnosed, juvenile diabetic boy sitting in the OPD diligently injecting himself with insulin which he removed from a small steel dabba. He had been trained by the nursing staff before he was discharged from the hospital and was a quick learner. He even went to the washroom to wash the small ball of cottonwool he had used to wipe off the needle! His mum worked at a nearby construction site and was clueless about the disease. She was frightened and wanted to know if her other children would contract the disease if they played with him. The boy was fighting back tears and so was I. Here was this brave little guy trying his best to cope with the pain of the needles (this was more than 20 years ago and the needles were not as fine as they are today, so they actually did hurt) and everything associated with the disease, and to top it all he had to hear what his mum had to say. My heart went out to him and I tried my very best to explain to her that his disease was not contagious, but because of the genetic factor she would have to get her younger children tested too. She grabbed his hand and walked out, muttering under her breath. I still say a prayer for him and hope he is doing well.

The beta cells of the islets of Langerhans of the pancreas make the hormone insulin. In a non- diabetic, whenever food is consumed, the beta cells release insulin to help the body use or store the blood glucose it gets from the carbohydrates present in the meal. IDDM or Type 1 diabetics have malfunctioning pancreas. The beta cells have been destroyed and hence no endogenous insulin is formed. These patients need shots of exogenous insulin in order to utilize the glucose from food. NIDDM or Type 2 diabetics do make endogenous insulin in their body. However, their body does not respond well to this endogenous insulin. If diet and exercise therapy fails, they may have to take oral hypoglycemic medications or shots of exogenous insulin in order to utilize the glucose from food. Shots of exogenous insulin cannot be swallowed like a pill because it would be broken down during digestion just like the protein in food. This exogenous insulin has to be injected into the fat under the skin for it enter into the blood stream. Injection sites have to be rotated for better response.

NIDDM or Type 2 diabetes is a progressive disease, and most patients will eventually need insulin to help them keep a tight control over their blood glucose levels and also to avoid complications associated with the disease. Research clearly shows that early and aggressive intervention to lower blood glucose levels reduces the risk of complications of the disease. Trying to delay taking insulin injections in uncontrolled diabetes is like flogging a dying horse to run a race—he can never win. It is therefore better to start insulin injections as soon as possible to prevent the early onset of diabetes-related complications than to lose an eye, a kidney, or a limb. Once the blood glucose levels are well controlled, most diabetologists will be happy to decrease the units of insulin dosage and to even do away with insulin injections altogether. However, it can be a daunting task for the doctors to decide which treatment regimen is appropriate to manage a particular patient. All Type 1 diabetics need insulin injections to keep blood glucose levels under control. Most doctors prescribe insulin injections for Type 2 diabetics when FBS levels are consistently more than 250 mg/dl or RBS levels are consistently more than 300 mg/dl or HbA1C is more than 10.

There are many different types of exogenous insulin. (1) **Rapid-acting exogenous insulin**, as the name suggests, works within fifteen minutes of injecting; its action peaks in an hour but continues to work for two to four hours. E.g., Lispro, Novolog, Humalog; (2) **Regular or short-acting exogenous insulin** works within thirty minutes of injecting; its action peaks within two to three hours but the action continues for three to six hours. E.g., Humulin R, Novolin R; (3) **Intermediate-acting exogenous insulin** works within two to four hours of injecting; its action peaks four to twelve hours later and continues for twelve to eighteen hours. E.g., Humulin N, Novolin N; (4) **Long-acting exogenous insulin** works several hours after injecting and its action continues for 24 hours. E.g., Lantus.

Exogenous insulin has three main characteristics: (1) Onset: it is the length of time before the injected exogenous insulin reaches the bloodstream and begins lowering the blood glucose level; (2) Peak action time: it is the time during which this exogenous insulin is at its maximum strength in order to lower the patient's blood glucose level; (3) Duration time: it is how long the exogenous insulin continues to lower the patient's blood glucose level.

Insulin vials should be be kept at temperatures ranging from 4–80 °C in the refrigerator. They should never be kept in the freezer. Pre-injection, the insulin vial should be brought down to body temperature by gently rubbing it between the palms of the hands. Only then should the insulin be withdrawn into the syringes. Keep the insulin vial at room temperature and away from heat and direct sunlight while travelling, in case refrigeration facilities are not available. Disposable syringes should be used. These can be reused about six to eight times by the same patient but never share needles with other patients. Change the needle once it gets blunt. The insulin injections are generally administered about 20–30 minutes prior to a meal. The needle must be inserted at a slight angle so that the injection is in the subcutaneous tissue; in overweight or obese patients with more subcutaneous fat, it would be correct to insert the needle vertically downwards. The sites where the injections can be given include the upper outer arms, upper outer thighs, lower abdomen, and buttocks. Injection sites need to be regularly rotated.

A patient needing exogenous insulin can opt for **injections from vials of exogenous insulin**, **pre-filled insulin pens,** and **insulin pumps**.

Inhaled, intranasal, and transdermal routes for delivery of exogenous insulin have met with poor response.

In a pre-filled insulin pen, a small pen-sized device holds an insulin cartridge which contains about 300 units of exogenous insulin. Cartridges are available in different insulin formulations. The amount of insulin to be injected is dialled in by turning the bottom of the pen until the required number of units is seen in the dose-viewing window. The tip of the pen consists of a needle that is replaced with each injection. A release mechanism allows the needle to penetrate just under the skin and deliver the required amount of insulin. The cartridges and needles are disposed of when finished and new ones simply are inserted. Many times, the entire pen is disposed of. The pre-filled insulin pen is less cumbersome than injections of insulin from glass vials.

An insulin pump is composed of a pump reservoir similar to that of an insulin cartridge, a battery-operated pump, and a computer chip that allows the user to control the exact amount of insulin being delivered. The pump is attached to a thin plastic tube (an infusion set) that has a cannula (like a needle but soft) at the end through which insulin passes. This cannula is inserted under the skin, usually on the abdomen. The cannula is changed every two days. The tubing can be disconnected from the pump while showering or swimming. The pump is used for continuous insulin delivery, 24 hours a day. The amount of insulin is programmed and administered at a constant rate (basal rate). Often, the amount of insulin needed over the course of 24 hours varies depending on factors like exercise, activity level, and sleep. The insulin pump allows for the user to programme many different basal rates to allow for this variation in lifestyle. In addition, the user can programme the pump to deliver additional insulin during meals to cover the excess demands for insulin caused by the ingestion of carbohydrates with the meal.

5

Controlling Diabetes With Diet

Once a diabetic realizes that the best way to keep a tight control over his blood glucose levels is through diet and exercise, he should not only keep a watch on what he eats and how much but also on when he eats. The best dietary regimen for a diabetic is one that enables him to keep his blood glucose, cholesterol, blood pressure, and weight within his target range, while allowing him to enjoy what he eats and not feel overly restricted. This would ensure that his compliance is maximum. Losing inches around the waistline is crucial when it comes to diabetes management. This is because belly fat gathers around the liver and the pancreas and damages the blood glucose regulatory mechanisms.

To successfully manage to keep a tight control over blood glucose levels, Type 2 diabetics need to make a commitment to lifestyle changes which include a healthy diet and an increase in physical activity, and stick to this commitment. The unconditional support of close family members will help the patient adhere to all the recommended treatment guidelines. These necessary changes can affect family members, since all family members are interdependent. Family plays a very important role in the health of each member, especially since healthy habits are often developed within the home. As long as the patient is supported by family members, he will be able to achieve his blood test targets. If, however, some members are not considerate and supportive, the diabetic will slip up and this can be detrimental to his health.

A healthy, balanced diet should be the backbone of glucose management for all patients diagnosed with diabetes. This type of a food regimen is tailor-made to include nutrients from the different food groups in the amounts and proportions required by that particular individual. A healthy, balanced diet also makes allowances for additional amounts of nutrients during periods of illness, deficiency, and injury. Fortunately or unfortunately, there is no one perfect food. In order to maintain good health, an assortment of nutrients are needed that can only be obtained by eating a wide variety of seasonal foods. Eating right is vital when a person is trying to prevent or control diabetes, especially if there is a family history of the disease.

Once the diagnosis of diabetes has been confirmed, most diabetics will resolve never to eat desserts again. So weeks 1, 2, and 3 go by without the consumption of any mithai, chocolate, sherbet, ice cream, etc. Even jaggery in the dal is banished from the dining table. Then it is time to test the blood glucose level again. Most of the time the blood glucose levels do not drop drastically and the patient gets puzzled and upset. What has he done wrong? What he has not realized is that all carbohydrate-rich foods finally get converted into glucose in the body. Glucose is the principal source of fuel for the body. So by not eating dessert and instead eating two more servings of dry bhakri or khakra or roti, he has not been able to achieve the desired blood glucose result.

Previously it was believed that a diabetic's diet should be different from what the rest of the family members were eating. Since glucose is derived from carbohydrates, diabetics were told to give up all carbohydrates and, instead, eat lots of protein and fat to meet their energy requirements. This was detrimental to their health because the increased protein intake put an additional load on the kidneys and the high-fat diet caused weight gain and cardiac disease. Other side effects included high blood pressure, gout, fatty liver, etc.

There is no longer any such thing as a 'diabetic diet'. The same dietary guidelines recommended for people in general, are recommended for people with diabetes. These guidelines include eating a wide variety of fresh fruit and vegetables; unrefined whole grains like jowar, bajra, ragi, barley, wheat, oats, rice, quinoa, etc.; complex carbohydrates from legumes, starchy vegetables, wholegrain breads and cereals; lean protein from low-fat paneer, edamame beans, or soy beans, eggs, chicken, fish, etc.; low-fat dairy products like skim milk, low-fat dahi, and paneer; healthful fats like those found in healthy olive and canola vegetable oils, seeds, nuts, low-fat fish, avocado, etc.; and fibre in appropriate portions.

Sugar is no longer strictly off a diabetic patient's food list as it previously was. Today, people with diabetes are allowed to eat 'desserts and sweets' in moderation as long as the sugar content is taken into consideration while formulating their diet plan. If they want to occasionally indulge in a small serving of dessert, they are encouraged to 'work' for it by 'working out'. A slice of fruit or a rasgulla that has the sugary syrup squeezed out of it still remain the best options whenever a diabetic wants to cater to his sweet tooth.

In spite of all these new dietary freedoms, many people with diabetes find it easier to follow prescriptive-type 'blood group diets' or 'gluten-free diets' or 'Glycemic Index food lists' or 'calorie charts' or 'exchange lists'. Over the years, I have seen that the more restrictions placed on a diabetic patient in terms of food control, the more likely they are to indulge in cheat meals and upset the blood glucose balance. This in turn leads to irritability, stress, and anger which further increases their levels. Therefore, I encourage them to do whatever it takes to keep their blood glucose levels under control. Adherence to basic dietary rules along with a spice mix tailormade to suit their health specifications results in better long-term management of diabetes.

Research now indicates that the best way to manage diabetes is to eat a balanced diet. The nutritional needs for a diabetic are virtually the same as for everyone else. A diabetic food plan is simply a healthy eating plan that is high in nutrients, low in fat, and moderate in calories. This is a healthy diet for anyone wishing to maintain good health always. A diabetic still needs to monitor his carbohydrate intake but the emphasis is now on the right kind of carbohydrate-rich foods.

The food we eat comprises macronutrients (carbohydrates, proteins, and fats) and micronutrients (vitamins and minerals). Macronutrients are needed in larger quantities and provide energy. Micronutrients are needed in smaller amounts and do not provide energy; however, they are essential for the proper functioning of the body. Carbohydrates and proteins each provide the body with 4 calories/gram but fats are calorie-dense and provide 9 calories/gram. Water is the most important nutrient that the body requires because all chemical reactions within the body take place in the presence of water. In fact, signals of thirst propel us to the nearest water fountain or water cooler before water levels in our body become dangerously low. Dehydration kills faster than starvation. Luckily, water is calorie-free!

DIABETIC DIETS AND CARBOHYDRATE INTAKE

These nutrients get converted into glucose after ingestion and digestion. This glucose is either used immediately for energy or is stored in the liver and muscle cells for future use. Carbohydrates play an important role in the body. They are the primary source of energy in the body, in the form of glucose. They help the body use proteins and fats in a proper manner. Proteins are needed for growth, to build muscle, and to repair worn-out tissues. Fats are needed, albeit in smaller amounts, to lubricate and maintain healthy cell walls, and they also play a role in cholesterol metabolism. In the absence of carbohydrate, the body uses protein as a source of energy and more fat is broken down than the body is equipped to handle. Carbohydrates are of different types. It is important to choose the right ones and in the correct amounts, in order to maintain a tight control on blood glucose levels and manage diabetes well. This in turn will stave off the onset of complications associated with uncontrolled diabetes.

Refined or simple carbohydrates comprise various forms of sugar or sucrose. Sucrose is made up of glucose and fructose or fruit sugar. Simple sugars include table sugar added to the morning cup of tea and also sugars present in refined foods like white bread, maida biscuits, jellybeans, cakes, pastries, candy, etc.

Unrefined or complex carbohydrates include fibres and starches such as those found in oats, wholemeal flours, legumes, potatoes, unpolished rice, multigrain bread, etc. Starch is found in grains, some fruits and vegetables, and nuts and seeds. It can be digested by the human body into its constituent glucose molecules. Fibre is a type of carbohydrate that cannot be digested by the human body. Yet it is essential to good health because it gives a feeling of fullness and also helps get rid of toxins. Both soluble as well as the insoluble forms of fibre are beneficial. Fibre is found in fruits and vegetables and in the outer layers of grains. Processed foods lack fibre.

There are two kinds of fibre found in food, depending on their ability to dissolve in water or not. **Insoluble fibre** is called roughage, e.g., bran, skins and seeds of fruits and vegetables, vegetables and cereal. This kind of fibre promotes regularity by adding bulk to the bowel movements and prevents constipation, slows digestion in order to help in weight loss and blood glucose control, and helps prevent intestinal disorders. Insoluble fibre also reduces the risk of intestinal cancers. **Soluble fibre** is that part of the plant material which absorbs water, and swells and dissolves in the digestive system. Oat bran, barley, legumes, and fruit are high in soluble fibre. This fibre also works to moderate blood glucose, reduce cholesterol and triglycerides, and lower LDL cholesterol. Thus fibre is a vital nutrient. Its recommended daily allowance is 20–35 gm per day. A diet rich in fibre and carbohydrate may decrease the postprandial rise in blood sugar and in serum insulin and help in keeping blood lipid levels under control.

Refined or processed sugary foods containing simple carbohydrates are often slotted in the same category as unrefined carbohydrates, leading people to believe that all carbohydrates cause weight gain. It is these highly processed foods which are depleted of fibre and nutrients that tend to give all carbohydrates a bad name. This results in carb-free or low-carb diets which can be fatal to a diabetic, especially one who is on allopathic medication. Carbohydrates are an essential part of the diabetic diet. Therefore, the diabetic diets should be viewed as regulated rather than restricted in terms of carbohydrate. Irrespective of whether one is a diabetic or not, a 100 per cent wholewheat slice of bread or a mixed-grain bhakri is a healthier option than a doughnut or a roomali roti made from maida (processed wheat flour).

Carbohydrates have a big impact on the blood glucose levels, much more than proteins and fats. However, carbohydrates do not have to be avoided when one is diagnosed with diabetes. Instead, smart choices have to be made. In general, it is best to limit the intake of refined carbohydrates like white bread, instant oats, regular pasta, white rice, aerated beverages, desserts, and highly salted and processed snacks. High-fibre complex carbohydrates called slow-release carbohydrates are a smarter option. They are digested more slowly, have more satiety value because they prolong the feeling of fullness, prevent the pancreas from producing too much insulin, and help keep the blood glucose levels even, rather than causing a glucose spike.

Choose	Instead of
brown rice, quinoa, couscous	white rice
sweet potatoes, mashed cauliflower, yam, tapioca	mashed potatoes
wholewheat pasta	regular pasta
wholewheat or wholegrain bread	white bread
bran flakes and high-fibre cereal	sugary cereal
slow-cooked oats	instant oats
bran muffin	regular muffin
wholegrain or multigrain roti	regular paratha
oatmeal uttapam	uttapam
mixed-grain idlis	idlis
mixed-seed hummus	regular hummus

Refined foods have a higher **glycemic index (GI)** while unrefined foods have a comparatively lower glycemic index. Glycemic means 'sugar in the blood'. The glycemic index is a numerical system of measurement that indicates how quickly a food converts into glucose in the body. Glucose has a GI of 100 and the GI list gives each food a rating between zero and 100. **Glycemic load (GL)** is a newer term that looks at both, the GI and the amount of carbohydrate in a food, giving a much more accurate idea of how a food affects the blood glucose level. High-GI foods spike the blood glucose while low-GI foods are safe to eat. The GI and GL rank all carbohydrate-rich foods on a scale that is based on their immediate effect on raising the blood glucose after they have been eaten. This is known as the **glycemic response of food**. Refined foods, cakes, pastries, white bread, boiled sweets and candies, cornflakes, etc. all have a high GL. Cereals and potatoes have a fibre content and yet have a comparatively high GI. The GI of a food is different when it is eaten alone than when it is eaten with another food. The way in which these foods are eaten also affects their GI.

For example, if cereals are eaten with milk (which contains protein) or potatoes are eaten with butter (which contains fat), the GI changes. The riper a fruit or vegetable, the higher its GI. Fruit juice, mashed potatoes, and soft-cooked vegetables have a higher GI than whole fruit, baked potatoes, and crunchy cooked veggies respectively. Since the GI–GL values for the same foods are not consistent, these values are a source of controversy.

High glycemic index: 70–100. Foods with a high GI have a tendency to increase blood glucose levels very rapidly. If the patient is also trying to reduce or maintain his weight then it is essential to avoid these foods completely. The pancreas releases large amounts of insulin when high-GI foods rapidly spike the blood glucose levels. If this glucose is not utilized immediately it will be stored as fat. E.g., ragi 98, maize 89, baked potato 85, cornflakes 83, bajra 82, whole green gram 81, coffee 79, instant porridge 79, Weetabix 77, waffles 76, doughnut 76, horse gram 73, watermelon 72, bagel 72, white bread 70.

Intermediate or medium glycemic index: 55–70. Foods with a medium GI have to be included in moderation in order to prevent weight gain and also spikes in blood glucose levels. E.g., sweet biscuits 69, croissant 67, sugar 65, couscous 65, chhole 63, barley 61, black gram 61, honey 58, digestive biscuits 58, white rice 58, basmati rice 58, popcorn 55, brown rice 55.

Low glycemic index: Below 55. In order to achieve weight loss and also to keep blood glucose levels within the normal range, it is always advisable to plan meals from this list of foods. Low-GI foods keep one fuller for a longer time and also help control appetite. E.g., burger bun 61, banana 55, green gram dal 54, kiwi 52, orange juice 52, wholegrain bread 50, slow-cooked porridge 49, baked beans 48, grapefruit juice 48, multigrain bread 48, noodles 47, pineapple juice 46, carrot juice 45, yoghurt 44, lentil soup 44, apple juice 41, pasta 41, besan atta 39, apples 36, soy milk 30, lentils 29, milk 27, kidney beans 27, channa dal 16, soy beans 16, broccoli 15, celery 15, cucumber 15.

Carbohydrates impact blood glucose levels hence understanding carbohydrates will go a long way in improving these levels. Foods with carbohydrates include:

- grains like rice, wheat, jowar, bajra, ragi, couscous, bread, pizza, pasta, roti, chapatti, paratha, biscuits, oats, cereals like wheat flakes, muesli, etc.
- starchy vegetables like potatoes, yam, tapioca, carrots, peas, corn;
- fruits like apple, mango, banana, kiwi, grapefruit, papaya, etc. and also fruit juices
- milk and milk products like dahi, mava, etc.
- sugars, honey, jaggery, desserts, mithai, etc.

DIABETIC DIETS AND FRUIT INTAKE

Carbohydrate in fruit, i.e., fructose and sucrose, causes the blood glucose level to increase. This increase is even more pronounced if fruit is eaten immediately after a carbohydrate-rich meal. However, fruit provides the body with vitamins, minerals, antioxidants and soluble as well as insoluble fibre. Therefore, a diabetic diet should always include a couple of servings of fruit even if the fruit is sweet. Instead of eating fruit along with or immediately after a meal, it should be eaten as a snack in between the consumption of two main meals. Fruit juices should be avoided because they are generally devoid of fibre and hence cannot retard the absorption of fructose in the body. Some fruit like mango and custard apple do contain more sugar than others, but diabetics with good blood glucose control can incorporate them in their diets as an in-between-meals carbohydrate snack.

One serving of fruit should ideally contain 15 gm of carbohydrates, i.e., 60 calories. The size of the serving depends on the carbohydrate content of the fruit. So the serving size of fruit like papaya and apple will be much larger than the serving size of fruit like mango and banana. The advantage of eating a low-carbohydrate fruit is that one can consume a larger portion. But irrespective of whether a low-carbohydrate or high-carbohydrate fruit is eaten as a snack, so long as the serving size provides 15 gm of carbohydrates, the effect on the blood sugar is the same.

The following fruit servings contain about 15 gm of carbohydrates:

1 medium-sized apple
½ medium banana
120 gm cherries
80 gm chickoo
½ medium-sized grapefruit
1 medium-sized katori grapes
1 medium-sized guava
1 kiwi
6 lychees
80 gm chopped mango
1 orange
140 gm papaya
1 medium-sized peach
1 medium-sized pear

100 gm chopped pineapple
3 plums
180 gm strawberries
1 sweet lime
200 gm chopped watermelon

Diabetic Diets and Protein Intake

Proteins are also macronutrients that provide energy. Each gram of protein provides 4 calories of energy. They make up half of the total body weight and are present in the muscles, bones, body fluids and secretions, blood, and skin. Proteins play an important role in the body. They are needed for growth in children and cell repair of worn-out tissues in adults. They build teeth, bones, skin, muscles, and blood. They strengthen the immune system, increase antibodies, and help the body fight diseases. Proteins are the main structural elements of the skin, muscles, skeletal tissue, connective tissue, nails, hair, and cell membranes. Proteins are made up of **amino acids** which are known as the building blocks of protein. Amino acids include **essential amino acids** and **non-essential amino acids**. Depending upon their amino acid content, proteins are classified as complete proteins, partially complete proteins and incomplete proteins. **Complete proteins** contain all the essential amino acids, e.g., animal proteins found in meat, fish, poultry, eggs, milk and milk products. They support life and promote growth. **Partially complete proteins** contain a combination of essential as well as non-essential amino acids, e.g., vegetarian sources of protein like that found in lentils, beans, grains, nuts, and seeds. They can only support life. **Incomplete proteins** contain non-essential amino acids and lack essential amino acids, e.g., protein present in gelatin. They neither support life nor promote growth.

Diabetics do not usually need any more protein than non-diabetics, and there are times, especially when kidney function is impaired, when less protein is better. As long as the kidneys are healthy and functioning well, about 15–20 per cent of the daily calories should come from protein. About 60–70 per cent of the calories should come from carbohydrates, especially complex carbohydrates, and the remainder should come from fat. Diabetic patients with kidney disease are asked to limit their protein intake to a maximum of 1 gram of protein per kg of body weight.

DIABETIC DIETS AND FAT INTAKE

Fats are also essential macronutrients. They are calorie-dense. Each gram of fat provides 9 calories of energy. They are needed to make hormones like estrogen, progesterone, and testosterone. Fats also help in the absorption of fat-soluble vitamins A, D, E, and K. They lubricate the joints, insulate nerve cells, improve suppleness of the skin, and impart warmth to the body. Fats are needed to stabilize cholesterol production and regulate the clotting of blood as well as blood pressure.

Fats like oil, mayonnaise, cream, butter, and avocado do not raise the blood glucose levels. In fact, fats slow down the rate at which the stomach empties, and decrease the rate at which the blood glucose level increases after a mixed meal. If fats are consumed in excess and are not utilized by the body for energy purposes then they are stored in the adipose cells and make up the adipose tissue.

The type of fat eaten has a bearing on the health of the

individual. Fats are classified as saturated fats, trans fats, monounsaturated fats, and polyunsaturated fats. Dietary fats or triglycerides are the fats in foods. Saturated fats found in meat, butter, lard, etc. raise LDL cholesterol levels, which is not desirable. Transaturated or hydrogenated fats, found in some margarine and vegetable shortenings, biscuits, crackers, cookies, etc. also raise LDL cholesterol levels. Hence their intake should be avoided. Monounsaturated fats found in avocado, nuts, canola oil, and olive oil can improve cholesterol ratios. Polyunsaturated fats found in soyabean oil, safflower oil, corn oil, fish oils, etc. also help lower blood cholesterol levels. Saturated fats are solid at room temperature whereas unsaturated fats are liquid at room temperature.

Cholesterol is a waxy, fat-like substance made in the liver, which is needed for the manufacture of bile acids, Vitamin D, and steroid hormones in the body. Dietary cholesterol is only found in non-vegetarian sources of food like meat, egg yolks, milk and milk products, shellfish, etc. Vegetarian sources of food like fruits, vegetables, nuts, seeds and oilseeds, grains, etc. are devoid of cholesterol.

DIABETIC DIETS AND CAFFEINE INTAKE

Research shows that there is a strong relationship between caffeine intake and blood glucose levels. Even a cup of black coffee, which is devoid of both milk and sugar, can slightly raise blood glucose levels. Although coffee has long been associated with reducing the risk of developing Type 2 diabetes, studies show that high doses of caffeine can increase the blood glucose levels by up to 8 per cent. This means that there are other components in caffeinated and decaffeinated coffee that can reduce the blood glucose levels but pure caffeine, in capsule form, raises glucose levels. This pure caffeine could perhaps alter the function of insulin or the surge of adrenaline or cortisol that accompanies the intake of large doses of caffeine, could be the reason why blood glucose levels increase.

Hence a diabetic, who is frustrated by his inability to control his ailment, would do well to check his coffee-drinking habit and keep it under control. Switching to decaffeinated coffee, which has chlorogenic acid and trigonelline, might help. Both chlorogenic acid and trigonelline were seen to have reduced the insulin and glucose response for a period of fifteen minutes after the ingestion of glucose in an oral glucose tolerance test (OGTT).

Tea, on the other hand, is a more widely used beverage than coffee, and has been used for medicinal purposes in many parts of the world for many years. Tea contains polyphenols which are chemicals that have anti-cancer, anti-inflammatory and antioxidant effects. These teas are the light brews without milk and sugar, and not the over brewed masala chai versions that so many Indians are addicted to. Tea also contains caffeine. Both green tea and oolong tea decrease blood glucose levels and improve HbA1C, total cholesterol, and LDL cholesterol levels. In fact, drinking green tea may lower the risk of developing Type 2 diabetes along with reducing blood pressure.

Teas have some side effects and interfere with nutrients and drug action if consumed in large or excessive quantities. Iron supplements are generally taken at breakfast. Tea may interfere with the absorption of iron from these supplements and also from food. So drinking tea after a meal rich in iron like methi–palak, or while taking an iron supplement at breakfast is not the smartest thing to do. Tea may also interfere with certain laboratory tests, thallium tests, uric acid tests, etc. Tea may also worsen glaucoma due to increase in eye pressure.

Drinking excessive amounts of both tea and coffee may cause insomnia, tremors, anxiety, and restlessness, and increased bleeding if used with blood thinners. However, limiting the intake of these beverages to two to three cups per day is permitted in a diabetic diet.

DIABETIC DIETS AND FAMILY SUPPORT

Whilst planning a diet for a patient with diabetes, I ask about how understanding and supportive the family members and friends are. This is because the support of loved ones plays a major role in diabetes care. Non-supportive family members and friends can derail a diabetic's diet plan and come in the way of helping him maintain a tight control over his blood glucose levels. Patients have shared stories of how, despite their best efforts, they have not really been able to adhere to dietary restrictions. They have narrated instances of how an aunt tempts them to eat 'just one more kalakand' because 'nothing will happen' or of how children throw tantrums if the Sunday lunch is not at their favourite biryani restaurant even though they know that their diabetic parent cannot resist the temptation of overeating the finger-licking good food there or of how friends force them to drink 'one last peg of whiskey for the road' or of how their mother will insist that they eat mithai 'because it is prasad'.

Supporting a loved one with diabetes can be challenging as well as overwhelming for the relative or friend as well as the diabetic patient. Non-diabetics need to understand everything about the disease so that they can be of better help and support in keeping the patient safe from diabetic complications. The most important thing to know is the warning signs and symptoms of hypoglycemia and hyperglycemia. Hypoglycemia occurs when blood glucose levels are too low. Hyperglycemia, on the other hand, occurs when blood glucose levels are too high. If a blood glucose monitor is not readily available at the time, the caregiver needs to be able to differentiate between the two and know what steps to take for both. In this way, diabetic complications can be averted.

What a diabetic can do alone to fight diabetes and its consequences, can be done so much more effectively together with loved ones. So if a family member or a close friend is diagnosed with diabetes you can help in the following ways:

- Accompany him to the next appointment with the diabetologist and nutritionist to learn from them how to help the patient.
- Understand from the doctor how the prescribed medications work and, more importantly, when they should be given and what their side effects are.
- Learn how to use the glucometer and also encourage the patient to monitor his blood glucose levels at regularly scheduled times. A random blood glucose test is OK occasionally, but it is always best to check after fasting for 8–10 hours and two hours after eating a main meal like breakfast, lunch, or dinner.
- Speak to the nutritionist about how best you can be of help to the patient by making the right food choices during the planning of meals and also at mealtime. Learn how to prepare healthy diabetic meals and snacks. This is because diet plays a major role in controlling the blood glucose levels.
- If the patient is a close family member/friend, you can carry

extra medication for them when going to a restaurant or a picnic or a party. This way, if the patient has forgotten his medication at home it would not lead to a blood sugar spike. Also, carry a small snack like a fruit or some khakra or crackers to prevent a dip in sugar if the meal is not served on time.

➢ Encourage the patient to exercise by joining him at the local gym, swimming pool, or garden. Some malls allow people to walk in their extensive lobbies and corridors as early as 6 am. So get there early, walk briskly for an hour, and maybe plan the day's meetings or catch up on some gossip whilst eating a wholesome breakfast post exercise.

➢ Follow-ups for check-ups with the healthcare team are extremely important. Encourage the patient to regularly fix an appointment with them, or better still, make the calls yourself.

➢ Be prepared to deal with the emotional situations that arise whenever there are spikes or dips in the blood glucose levels. Support the patient emotionally when she/he experiences fear, anxiety, depression, and loss of morale.

➢ It is equally important for you to watch yourself so that you do not become overwhelmed with caregiver stress. This can take a toll on your mental and physical health and well-being. So take a short break, rejuvenate, and come back better equipped to handle any diabetic emergencies.

DIABETIC DIETS AND THE YOUNG DIABETIC CHILD

A young diabetic child has to be made to understand that in order to maintain good blood glucose control, he will have to learn to eat healthy. Every growing child needs a healthy, balanced diet which includes nutrients from the different food groups. Parents are often at their wits' end while trying to meet the nutritional needs of their child; a diabetic child's diet needs a little more care and planning. The adjustment can be difficult for the diabetic child and for the rest of the family, whose unconditional love and support are crucial at all times.

The best thing to do would be to sit with the child's diabetologist and understand how many calories are being prescribed. Then get help from a nutritionist to convert the prescribed number of calories into a daily meal plan. Draw up a shopping list of a wide variety of foods from the different food groups, encourage the child to make healthy choices, and always keep plenty of healthy snack options readily available. Wholesome meals should be cooked for, and eaten by, all members of the family to encourage the diabetic child in his blood glucose battle.

A little extra effort will go a long way in helping a diabetic child live a normal life. Choose grilled, low-fat options when eating out. Encourage the child to increase his duration of exercise the day he wants to indulge in a small portion of dessert. When the child is invited to a birthday party, call the parent hosting the party to find out the menu and also to let her/him know that your child is diabetic and should not be forced to overeat. Pack a healthy snack—the hostess/host will definitely not mind. Monitor the child's blood glucose level before he leaves and give extra insulin if needed. This way the child will not have to miss out on little treats, as long as he is well prepared for it. Most importantly, the diabetic child should be taught to recognize the symptoms of hypoglycemia as well as those of hyperglycemia.

DIABETIC DIETS AND THE GENERAL GUIDELINES FOR BLOOD GLUCOSE CONTROL

- Rather than eating three large meals a day, a person, whether diabetic or not, would benefit from eating six to seven smaller meals in a day. This spacing out of the meals, at two- to three-hourly intervals, allows the pancreas to function better and release optimum amounts of the hormone insulin needed for better blood glucose management. Diabetics should eat breakfast within thirty minutes to one hour of waking up, eat a small amount of carbohydrates every two to three hours, and stop eating at least three hours before bedtime. This pattern of eating increases BMR (Basal Metabolic Rate), improves pancreatic function, increases energy levels, and decreases appetite. If, however, due to job constraints, a snack meal is not possible in between two main meals, a couple of nuts and seeds will also do.

- A diabetic patient should never skip breakfast. It is impossible to achieve blood glucose control by skipping the most important meal of the day—breakfast. It is easy to skip this main meal and the excuses to do so are many: time constraint, loss of appetite, the need to lose weight, glucose levels being too high, etc. Skipping breakfast can result in weight gain and, surprisingly, a further rise in blood glucose levels. A high-fasting blood glucose level does not always reflect what was eaten for dinner the previous night. It may very well have to do with the way in which the liver functions. The stores of glycogen in the liver are released into the blood at night, during sleep when food is not being consumed, to provide fuel. This works well for a non-diabetic person. In Type 2 diabetes, the liver is not able to realize that there is already a high level of glucose in the blood and may continue to release glycogen despite this. Eating a carbohydrate-rich meal like two idlis or a small serving of upma, poha, muesli, oatmeal, or two toasts at breakfast signals the liver to stop this release. This results in better blood glucose control throughout the day.

➢ Just as medication is to be taken at around the same time every day, a diabetic would benefit if he ate his three small main meals and three to four in-between snacks at around the same time every day. This is because eating meals throughout the day at roughly the same time each day provides a consistent source of energy or fuel. Also, the efficacy of the medication will be improved if this pattern is consistently maintained. The constant sway from energy highs to energy lows can also be avoided in this manner. This in turn will lead to less fatigue as well as a decrease in mood swings, depression and anxiety.

➢ Avoid eating mindlessly. It is important to be mindful of what is being eaten, and to keep a track on its effect on the blood glucose by testing before and after meals. The practice of mindfulness, that is, deliberately paying attention to the food being eaten, enables a person to learn to be aware of their physical hunger, differentiate this physical hunger from emotional or stress hunger, and eat until there is satiety by allowing the senses to fully relish every bite, be satisfied with eating less, and thoroughly enjoy the eating experience.

➢ Each of the six to seven meals should have some amount of carbohydrate to provide glucose and to keep the energy levels up and protein to ensure satiety or a feeling of fullness. Some good carbohydrate and protein combination options include:

For small main meals:
   A bowl of dal and rice khichdi and kadhi
   A bowl of fada-ni-khichdi with a glass of buttermilk
   A bowl of rice and rajma or chhole
   A bowl of couscous with steamed fish
   A bowl of quinoa with mushrooms
   A bowl of wholewheat pasta with steamed chicken
   A bowl of butter bean soup with 1 multigrain bread roll
   A bowl of mixed lentil and barley shorba
   2 mixed-grain rotis with low-fat paneer
   2 brown rice idlis with sambhar or dahi

For in-between snack meals:
   2 small green moong chilas with dahi
   3–4 pieces of dhokla with green chutney
   ½ cup carrot sticks with garlic hung curd dip
   A brown bread sandwich with a slice of low-fat cheese
   A bowl of pumpkin soup with 1 toast
   1 ragi khakra with 2 tablespoons hummus
   2 rice crackers with 1 tablespoon peanut butter
   1 small apple with 2 walnuts and 5 almonds
   2 low-fat paneer tikkis with 2 small baked puris
   1 pita pocket with rajma salad

DIABETES DIETS AND DINING OUT

In today's fast-paced world, people have no time to spend an entire day with family and friends. Gone are the days when people would plan one-day picnics, weekend drives to a nearby hill station, and so on and yummy homemade food would be lovingly packed in huge 'food cases' which jostled with suitcases for dicky space! People still want to de-stress, socialize, network, and meet family, friends, and business associates, albeit for a shorter time period. So dining out, ordering in, takeaway food parcels, a breakfast meeting with a client at the local south Indian restaurant, a quick coffee morning with the mothers of children's classmates have all become the order of the day.

Here are some tips to make eating out guilt-free and not cause havoc on blood glucose levels:

- Always try and choose a restaurant that provides a wide variety of food choices. This way, everyone at the table will be able to order their favourite food and not feel deprived.
- When ordering soups, steer clear of thick, creamy soups and chowders. Opt for clear broths like miso broth, egg drop soup, lemon grass chicken soup, tom yum soup, mushroom broth, minestrone, su-udon or noodle soup, wonton soup, gazpacho, lentil soup, and mixed vegetable or chicken consommé.
- At a fast-food restaurant, choose the skinless grilled fish or chicken and ask for a simple salad instead of fries. Make a request for the meat or fish to be poached, broiled, oven-baked, or grilled. If the fish or chicken is breaded or batter-fried and you have no other option, either send it back or remove the outer fried coating and just eat the meat.
- When ordering salads ask for the dressing to be served on the side, unless the dressing is lemon juice, a dash of olive oil, and vinegar. Pesto and arugula salad, Greek salad, Pad Thai salad, the simple tossed green salad, and even the

kachumber are great choices. Rich, creamy ranch dressings, mayonnaise, etc. are all high in fat and negate the health benefits of a garden-fresh, crunchy salad.

- Ask the server if unsure about the ingredients in a dish or the method of preparation. Most fine dining restaurants have a tagline to the dish, so read it carefully and remember that crispy, crunchy, and tempura all mean that the ingredients have been dipped in a flour- and/or egg-based batter and then deep-fried. When a baked dish is 'au gratin', it generally means that it is topped with cheese, so ask the chef to hold on to the cheese and instead use breadcrumbs to give that golden-brown colour.
- Tandoori rotis, tandoori paneer, veggies, and meats are healthier than cream- and oil-filled gravy dishes. But remember to ask the chef not to apply butter/ghee/oil to the food item once it is removed from the tandoor. Steamed brown rice and dal without tadka can also be ordered while steering clear of the maa ki dal, chhole, and rajma.
- At a south Indian restaurant order the Andhra tomato rice, the south Indian kadhi, piping-hot rasam with steamed rice or fluffy idlis, mixed vegetable avial, pesarattu which is similar to a moong dal chila, Chettinad chicken, and lemon rice. Make a request for the food to have as little oil as possible.
- When ordering pasta, stay away from heavy cream-based white sauces and opt for tomato or marinara sauce. Spaghetti aglio e olio (with garlic and olive oil) is your safest bet. Politely request the chef to be frugal with the olive oil and to avoid the cheese in any Italian food preparation. The same goes for pizza. If the chef is willing to replace cheese with crumbled paneer, go for it!

- Many types of Asian foods are healthy when served authentically—cooked with very little or no oil, heavy on the veggies and light on fried meats. Chinese and Japanese dishes can be healthy as long as the meats and veggies are not deep-fried before being added to the sauce or gravy. Opt for steamed or stir-fried meats and veggies. Avoid the ubiquitous fried rice which is super-unhealthy. At a Japanese restaurant, ask for the food to be cooked in broth or rice wine instead of oil. Avoid the deep-fried 'pot-stickers'. Share the shabu-shabu which is a community broth pot in which meat and veggies can be cooked. Maki sushi, salmon, and tuna sashimi with wasabi, soy, mirin, and rice wine vinegar are also good choices.
- If the portion size is large, share the meal or first halve it and ask for one half to be packed to take home. Eat slowly and do not feel the need to eat everything that is on the plate just because it has been paid for. Eat the same amount that you generally eat at home or eat a smaller portion.
- Ask the chef to add very little salt and to serve all accompaniments like salad dressings, butter, sauces, and gravies on the side. This way you can opt for a smaller serving of the accompaniments and not have the comparatively healthier main course smothered in unhealthy fats.
- Many restaurants now offer the nutritional information of their menu items on their website. Before going to the restaurant, log on to their website and pre-plan your order based on the calorie and carbohydrate content. This way you are more likely to adhere to your dietary restrictions and meet your goals.

DIABETIC DIETS AND PORTION CONTROL

It is not just what the diabetic eats that can assist in keeping a tight control on the blood glucose levels. How much he eats is also very important to achieve this. If a diabetic patient is new to watching portion sizes, he may be worried about incorrectly estimating the amount of food he needs to keep his blood glucose levels as near to normal as possible. Weighing and measuring food all the time can help control weight and blood glucose, but it can be time-consuming and inconvenient. Approximating the portion size by comparing the food to common objects can make the process of portion control a lot simpler, thereby making diabetes management easier. Here are some ideas to help the diabetic with portion control and blood glucose management:

➤ Invest in a set of measuring spoons and measuring cups and glasses. They come in handy when measuring salad dressings, sauces, gravies as well as dalia, rice, upma, poha, vegetables, dals, soups, and beverages.

➤ A small food scale will give a more accurate measure of the food being eaten. Some chopping boards now have an in-built weighing scale at one corner.

➤ A cup of non-starchy vegetables like cucumber, lettuce, spinach, cauliflower, and cabbage is generally the size of a cricket ball, has 5 gm carbohydrates, 2 gm protein, and no fat.

➤ A medium-sized potato or sweet potato is roughly the size of a computer mouse, has 25 gm carbohydrate, 5 gm protein, and no fat.

➤ A cup of cooked corn or oats also has approximately the same nutrient value as that of potato.

- A cup of breakfast cereal is approximately the size of a fist, has 18 gm carbohydrates, 4 gm protein, and 2 gm fat.
- 1 cup of cooked rice or pasta or upma or poha has 15 gm carbohydrates and 3 gm protein. The fat content depends on how much has been added while cooking.
- A 90 gm portion of meat or fish is equivalent to the size of a deck of cards, has no carbohydrates, 21 gm protein, and the fat content (up to 20 gm) depends on how lean the meat is.
- A tablespoon of peanut butter has no carbohydrates, 7 gm protein, and 8 gm fat.
- At a buffet, either use a small/quarter/side plate to eat dinner from or half-fill the plate with salad greens and then take the carbohydrates and protein foods.
- Even if opting for packets of 'diet' bhujia, chivda, or crisps, it is better to divide the packet into smaller servings using a measuring cup and put each serving into a small Ziploc pouch. This will now become your very own single-serve snack option to eat on the go!
- Repeat the above process for 'diet' gelato and ice cream but remember to use a small snack box instead of a pouch and to store the boxes in the freezer section of your refrigerator!

Diabetic Diets and Alcohol Consumption

I am often asked by my diabetic patients who like their wine, champagne, single malt, and beer if they can continue to consume alcohol and, if yes, how much can they have without it affecting their health. If the spouse (either husband or wife) is a part of this conversation, then, depending upon the dynamics at home, the spouse will vehemently make their displeasure

Blood Sugar and Spice

loud and clear or will meekly roll their eyes and implore me to convince the patient to abstain. Next comes the discussion of how many pegs, the size of the pegs, and, most importantly, how many times a week. Most people are well aware that food has an impact on blood glucose levels but they have absolutely no clue of how alcohol affects blood glucose metabolism.

When alcohol is consumed, it does not get metabolized in the stomach. Instead, it quickly moves into the bloodstream and within five minutes of guzzling a bottle of beer or downing a vodka shot, there is sufficient amount of alcohol in the bloodstream which can be measured. The liver is the organ where alcohol metabolism takes place and it generally takes two hours to metabolize a single unit of alcohol. So at a party, if pegs of alcohol are being consumed much faster than the liver can metabolize the alchohol, then the alcohol quickly moves to the brain and other organs via the bloodstream. This results in the 'high' or 'buzz' that is often felt post alcohol consumption. It 'hits' to a greater extent if alcohol is consumed right after a three-day or seven-day liver detox.

If a diabetic patient is on insulin or on any oral hypoglycemic medications that stimulate the pancreas to produce more insulin like sulfonylureas, then alcohol should strictly *not* be consumed. The blood glucose levels can fall dangerously low post alcohol consumption. The reason for this hypoglycemia is that instead of regulating the blood glucose levels, the liver is busy removing alcohol from the bloodstream. The symptoms of too much alcohol in the bloodstream and symptoms of low blood glucose levels can be very similar: dizziness and light-headedness, disorientation, sleepiness, slurring of speech, tremors and shakiness, and the inability to hold an object properly. It is so easy for others to mistakenly confuse hypoglycemia for drunkenness. A case that comes to mind is that of a diabetic who went into hypoglycemia whilst boarding an international flight. Not only was he offloaded but he was also thrown out of the airport because airline staff thought that he was drunk. Alcohol and diabetes are another reminder that it is always a good idea to wear an ID card that reads 'DIABETIC'.

Consuming alcohol can worsen complications associated with diabetes like high blood pressure, kidney damage and kidney failure, liver damage, eye damage, and peripheral nerve damage. Alcohol should also not be consumed if the patient has a history of alcohol abuse, has hypertriglyceridaemia or pancreatitis, is planning to conceive a child, is pregnant or lactating, or has a history of hypoglycemia. Alcohol reduces the normal rise of a diabetic patient's blood glucose in the early-morning hours. It also slows down or impairs both mental as well as physical abilities.

If the blood glucose levels are being managed well and are in good control, a small amount of alcohol is allowed, but not more than 2 units a day for men and not more than 1 unit a day for women. 1 unit of alcohol is the equivalent of 25 ml of whisky, vodka, or gin; 50 ml of sherry; and half a pint of medium-strength beer or lager. A serving of alcohol is equivalent to 1.5 oz of distilled spirits like whisky, rum and vodka; 5 oz of wine; or 12 oz of beer. Moderate alcohol intake does have some health benefits with respect to the heart and the blood vessels. So a diabetic is allowed to indulge in small amounts of alcohol only if the diabetologist allows it and the nutritionist can incorporate it into the meal plan after adjusting the calories.

Binge drinking and drinking alcohol on an empty

stomach or without monitoring blood glucose levels can all be detrimental to good health. Food serves as a buffer and slows down the absorption of alcohol in the bloodstream. Hence it is better to drink small amounts of alcohol preferably along with or after a meal. Blood glucose levels should be monitored after alcohol consumption, especially at night before going to bed. It is best to carry along a source of simple sugar if the blood glucose levels start to fall. Consuming alcohol after a workout can also be dangerous because the combination of the two will increase the chances of developing hypoglycemia.

DIABETIC DIETS AND HYPOGLYCEMIA

Hypoglycemia, signified by low blood glucose levels, is a scary side effect of diabetes that requires immediate action and proper treatment. When a diabetic patient begins experiencing symptoms of a dip in the blood glucose levels, he should take steps to increase his levels. If this is not treated promptly and properly, hypoglycemia can result in fits or seizures, sudden loss of consciousness, coma, permanent damage to the central nervous system, and even death. Being prepared and knowing what to do in case of hypoglycemia is an important part of a good diabetes management plan. For this reason, all diabetics should have a badge or wrist band or key ring that identifies them as diabetic.

Patients on insulin or oral hypoglycemic agents should be aware of hypoglycemia symptoms. These vary from person to person and also from episode to episode in the same person. These symptoms generally include:

- sudden or gradual drop in energy levels
- weakness and fatigue

- sleepiness
- inability to think clearly, confusion, fuzziness and delirium
- headaches
- dizziness and light-headedness
- blurring of vision
- tremors and shakiness, inability to hold an object
- palpitations, nervousness and a sudden sinking feeling
- cold sweats even while in an air-conditioned room, clammy skin
- difficulty in speaking and making others comprehend what is happening
- extreme hunger

Since hypoglycemia can cause loss of consciousness, if the diabetic patient is driving he should immediately pull over; if descending stairs or walking, he should sit down; if handling heavy machinery, he should alert his co-workers so as to not cause any harm to himself as well as to others.

Next, it is important to use a glucometer to test if it actually is an episode of hypoglycemia. My driver took his diabetic mum to a local healthcare centre when she was experiencing dizziness. Despite knowing that she was diabetic, the staff there put her on glucose intravenously without first checking her blood glucose levels. Later the family found out that her BP had fallen, not her blood glucose level. When the doctor checked an hour later, her RBS level had crossed 450 mg/dl. Quick action needs to be taken if the levels fall below 70mg/dl.

A diabetic experiencing hypoglycemia should quickly ingest carbohydrates in the form of fast-release simple sugars. The key to treating this condition is to be prepared at all times, especially if on insulin or oral hypoglycemic agents. Always keep a couple of toffees handy. Other foods that can quickly raise the blood glucose levels include 3–4 crackers, 2–3 cream-centre biscuits, 12–15 raisins, a cup of milk, a few sips of fruit juice or aerated beverage, a marble-sized lump of jaggery, a tablespoon of honey or of sugar, or a piece of mithai.

Do not overeat any of this as the blood glucose levels may go too high and result in hyperglycemia. Instead, wait for fifteen to 20 minutes and test again. If still low, eat more and repeat till the blood glucose levels rise and cross the 70mg/dl mark. If, however, the body does not respond, the patient should be rushed to the hospital by family members or colleagues at work. Here, the line of treatment is usually injections of glucagon which cause the blood glucose levels to rise immediately.

If these episodes of hypoglycemia are a regular feature, the patient needs to discuss medication adjustment with his doctor and meal plan adjustment with his nutritionist. Also take steps to ensure that their instructions are properly followed. Often a long-term patient of diabetes, especially one on insulin, feels quite confident about adjusting his dosage of insulin injection depending on his last blood glucose reading or on the menu for his next meal. The effect of this can sometimes be fatal.

DIABETIC DIETS AND SUGAR SUBSTITUTES

Refined sugar is high in 'empty' calories because it has no nutritional value, that is, it has no protein, no fat, no vitamins, and no minerals. In fact, when sugar is consumed, minerals like calcium, sodium, potassium, and magnesium are taken from various parts of the body to make use of this ingested sugar. Often, so much calcium is used to neutralize the effects of sugar that the bones become osteoporotic due to the large amounts of calcium withdrawn from the bones.

Sugar consumption can lead to weight gain which in turn can increase the risk for developing diabetes. Fruit sugar or fructose and its derivative, high-fructose corn syrup can help swimmers and other athletes boost their performance because they do not have to be broken down and go directly into the liver. As for non-athletes, the consumption will lead to obesity, increase in serum triglyceride levels, increase in HDL levels, decrease in LDL levels, increase in uric acid levels, spike in blood glucose levels, non-alcoholic fatty liver disease, dental caries, depression, yeast infections, acne, risk of cancer ... the list is endless and just goes on to show that sugar is a 'sweet best friend secretly plotting our early meeting with our Creator'. This is scary because sugar is present in almost all processed foods be it colas, iced teas, fruit and vegetable juices, sports drinks, chips, crackers, biscuits, energy bars, bhujia, chivda and other snack foods, cheese spread, jams, table spreads, peanut butter, ketchup, dips, sauces, and even in infant formula! So even if you avoid adding table sugar to tea and coffee, it is stealthily getting into your system and slowly poisoning you.

With all these harmful side effects associated with refined sugar and high-fructose corn syrup (HFCS), I am often asked if there is anything safe to use to sweeten foods and beverages. There are so many sugar substitutes readily available in the market that regular sugar seems to be moving right out of the local bania's shelf. Walk into any home or office and when you are offered a cup of tea, the little box of sugar substitute is jostling for tray space with the sugar bowl and the gur-shakkar bowl. A sugar substitute is a food additive that tastes like ... sugar. But are these safe or will they do more harm than good? This is certainly a good question. Exercise caution when choosing an alternative, because many sugar substitutes that are widely regarded as good for health are anything but healthy in reality.

Sugar substitutes include artificial sweeteners, natural sweeteners, sugar alcohols, and dietary sugar supplements. For those watching their weight or trying to lose some, these low-calorie or zero-calorie substitutes seem like a good thing. For diabetics, sugar substitutes do not cause as dramatic spikes in blood glucose levels as compared to sugar. Yet sugar substitutes can be much more harmful than *small* amounts of sugar and fructose. They can cause greater weight gain and increased hunger than regular table sugar. I will discuss each of these sugar substitutes. Whether you choose natural, artificial, or conventional sweeteners is up to you. Do read and then make an informed choice.

Artificial Sweeteners: include **aspartame** (Equal, NutraSweet, Spoonful, Indulge,) **sucralose** (Splenda), **saccharin** (Sweet'N Low), **acesulfame potassium** (Sunett, Sweet One), and **neotame** (Sweetos). Now there is a new hybrid sweetener called tagatose that is natural and has fewer calories than sugar. Research shows that there are many harmful effects associated with the use of artificial sweeteners and so their use should be avoided like the plague. Since these sweeteners are made from potentially toxic chemicals, their dangers continue to generate research, news coverage, and even more confusion in the minds of the consumers. The FDA (US Food and Drug Administration) says they are safe but there are health-conscious groups who aver that the research on artificial sweeteners is skewed and does not take into account the health impact on long-term usage.

➢ **Aspartame**: The dubious honour of being the most harmful of the lot of artificial sweeteners goes to aspartame.

Since it worsens insulin sensitivity, aspartame should *not* be used by diabetic patients. Aspartame is 200 times sweeter than sugar. It actually contains 4 calories per gm, but since so little is used there are only trace calories per serving. Aspartame is extremely harmful for patients with phenylketonuria (PKU) because aspartame has phenylalanine. It can decrease IQ, and cause mental retardation and behavioural problems. The methanol in aspartame, when metabolized, converts into formaldehyde, a substance used to embalm the dead! Remember the laboratory specimens in your biology lab? Traces of this formaldehyde were found in the kidney, liver, and brain of test subjects who were consuming aspartame.

There are over ninety-two different side effects on the health of an individual associated with using aspartame on a regular basis. These include bulging of eyes, blurring of vision, decreased vision, blindness, severe headaches and migraines, loss of memory, confusion, fatigue, fibromyalgia, tinnitus, noise intolerance and hearing impairment, dizziness, tremors, numbness of limbs, incoherent speech, anxiety, mood swings, depression, PMS (premenstrual syndrome), palpitation, breathlessness, elevated blood pressure, nausea, diarrhoea, ulcers, bloating, hives, improper control on blood glucose levels, hypoglycemia … the list is frighteningly endless.

- **Sucralose**: It is a chlorinated artificial sweetener like aspartame and saccharin, and just as bad for health. Sucralose is more chemically similar to DDT than it is to sugar and everybody knows exactly how toxic DDT is. Sucralose is found in a wide array of food products such as baked goods, non-alcoholic beverages, chewing gum, frozen dairy desserts, fruit juice, etc. It halves the amount of good bacteria in the intestines, makes the body more alkaline by increasing the pH level in the intestines, causes gastrointestinal issues, bloating and weight gain, breathlessness, allergies, sneezing, rashes, hives and itchy skin, severe headaches and migraines, dizzy spells, spikes in blood glucose levels, joint pain, palpitations, nausea and vomiting, diarrhoea, anxiety and depression. Sucralose can also shrink the thymus gland, an immune-system regulator. Pretty scary information that is enough to make you read food labels more carefully.

- **Saccharin**: In 1878 a researcher, Constantin Fahlberg, working on coal-tar derivatives in Baltimore, first discovered saccharin. It is a chlorinated artificial sweetener like aspartame and sucralose. Saccharin is 200–700 times sweeter than sugar but unlike sugar, it does not raise blood glucose levels. It has zero calories like other non-nutritive sweeteners. It is used in toothpaste, medicines, cookies, biscuits and other sugar-free bakery products, aerated beverages, chewing gum, breath mints and mouth washes. When consumed in large amounts it leaves a bitter, metallic aftertaste. Since it is very sweet to taste, it triggers the release of insulin and can lead to hypoglycemia in diabetics. Studies on laboratory rats showed that it could cause bladder cancer. These studies were not conclusive for human beings. Saccharin, however, should not be consumed by pregnant women, women who are breastfeeding, infants, and children as it causes allergic reactions.

- **Acesulfame potassium or Acesulfame-K**: It contains methylene chloride, a known carcinogen that can cause nausea, headaches, mood swings, depression, liver and kidney damage, problems with eyesight, and possibly cancer. Acesulfame-K can also lead to hypoglycemia in diabetics because its sweet taste triggers the release of insulin. Acesulfame-K is 200 times sweeter than table sugar, as sweet as aspartame, about two-thirds as sweet as saccharin, and one-third as sweet as sucralose. Like saccharin, it has a slightly bitter, metallic aftertaste, especially when ingested in large amounts. It is used in bakery foods, aerated beverages, and pharmaceutical products to mask the taste of the active medical ingredient and make it more palatable.

- **Neotame**: It is 13,000 times sweeter than table sugar, and about thirty times sweeter than aspartame, making it possibly an even more potent and dangerous neurotoxin and immunotoxin than aspartame, that can lead to cell death. Since studies are still being carried out, we will have to wait and watch. Until then it is best to avoid it if you are concerned about your health and that of your family.
- **Natural sweeteners**: Apart from honey, none of the natural sweeteners are readily available in our supermarkets and grocery stores. However, with more and more Indians travelling all around the world, they are willing to buy anything that remotely improves their health. If they themselves are not travelling, they will ask a well-meaning friend or relative to buy it for them or even order it from an online portal.

Natural sweeteners such as honey, molasses, maple syrup, and agave nectar may seem like a healthier choice, but they are loaded with fructose and some of them are also highly processed. The fact of the matter remains that sugar is sugar and too much sugar—whether it is *natural* or not—can adversely impact health. Even natural sweeteners are not a major source of vitamins and minerals. In these stressful times there is nothing wrong with the sweetness that a *little* sugar can bring to your life. So go ahead and indulge in the good stuff ... just remember to stop after eating a wee bit!

Some natural sweeteners include:

- **Honey**, made by bees from the nectar of flowers, is a ready-made sweetener that contains traces of nutrients. Honey is high in fructose, in fact 53 per cent of it *is* fructose. In its raw form, honey is completely natural. When used in moderation, raw honey has many health benefits.
- **Blackstrap molasses** is made from the third boiling of the sugar syrup and is the most nutritious molasses, containing substantial amounts of minerals like calcium, magnesium, potassium, and iron. It has a very strong flavour.
- **Rapadura** is the Portuguese name for unrefined dried sugarcane juice made simply by cooking sugarcane juice until it is very concentrated, and then drying it. This dried mass is then granulated or sold in the form of a block. It contains Vitamin C and iron. It can be used in baked goods like chocolate cake, brownies, coffee, and black tea. It is similar to our **sugarcane jaggery** and to the Spanish **panela**.
- **Turbinado sugar** is made by boiling sugarcane juice, cooling this, and then crystallizing it into granules. These granules are then refined to a light tan colour by removing impurities and surface molasses. A popular brand name of turbinado sugar is **Sugar in the Raw**, which can be found in most natural food stores.
- **Agave nectar** is produced from the juice of the core of the

succulent agave plant native to Mexico. This is the same plant used to make tequila! Agave nectar is sweeter and a little less viscous than honey. It contains trace amounts of iron, calcium, potassium, and magnesium. While high-fructose corn syrup contains 55 per cent fructose, agave nectar syrup contains 90 per cent fructose. Despite this, agave nectar has a **low glycemic index** because of its low glucose content. So diabetics can use small amounts of this natural sweetener as it does not cause the highs and lows that come with sugar and high-fructose corn syrup.

- **Brown rice syrup** is made when cooked white rice (not brown rice) is cultured with enzymes, which break down the starch in the rice. The resulting liquid is cooked and reduced to a thick syrup, which is about half as sweet as white sugar and has a mild butterscotch flavour. Brown rice syrup is composed of about 50 per cent complex carbohydrates, which break down more slowly in the bloodstream than simple carbohydrates, resulting in a less dramatic spike in blood glucose levels. Brown rice syrup has the tendency to make food harder and crispier, so it is great in crisps, granolas, and cookies.
- **Maple syrup** is often eaten with pancakes, waffles, French toast, or oatmeal and porridge. It comes from the sap of sugar maple, red maple, or black maple trees found in Canada and the United States. This sap is collected, filtered, and boiled down to make an extremely sweet syrup with a distinctive flavour. It contains fewer calories and a higher concentration of minerals like manganese and zinc than honey. It also has iron, potassium, and calcium albeit in smaller amounts. 'Maple-flavoured syrups' are imitations of real maple syrup. While true maple syrup contains

nothing but 'maple syrup', imitation syrups are made of high-fructose corn syrup, sugar, artificial sweeteners, and just 3 per cent of maple syrup.

> **Sugar alcohols**, commonly known as polyols, are carbohydrates that occur naturally in many fruits and vegetables that are eaten on a daily basis. They have fewer calories than table sugar and are more slowly absorbed and converted into glucose in the bloodstream. They do raise blood glucose levels after a meal, but not as high as table sugar does. They include **sorbitol, maltitol, mannitol, xylitol, lactitol, erythritol, glycerol, glucitol, and isomalt**. The next time you read a nutrient label on a packaged food product, the chances of finding one or more of these sugar alcohols is high. Polyols are used in the making of sugar-free candies, breath mints and lozenges, chewing gum, mouthwash, desserts, bakery products, chocolate, and ice creams. Cough syrups, chewable vitamins, and mineral supplements can also contain sugar alcohols.

Sugar alcohols provide fewer calories than table sugar because they are not completely absorbed into the body. The negative effect of this is that eating too many foods containing sugar alcohols can lead to abdominal gas and diarrhoea. Also **maltitol**, a commonly used sugar alcohol, spikes blood glucose levels almost as much as a starchy carbohydrate like yam or potato.

On the other hand, **xylitol,** made from corncobs, which looks like sugar, tastes like sugar, has the same sweetness as sugar, may be a better choice as a sugar substitute. Being a natural insulin stabilizer, it does not cause that great a spike in the blood glucose levels and also fights tooth decay. It helps reduce sugar and carbohydrate cravings. Keep it away from house pets because it can be poisonous to them.

Dietary Sugar Supplements include Stevia, Monk Fruit or Lo Han Guo and Pure Glucose (Dextrose)

Stevia is a highly sweet herb derived from the leaf of the North and South American stevia plant. Since it is 300 times sweeter than sugar, it is purified and sold as a dietary sugar supplement. Stevia is completely safe in its natural form and can be used to sweeten most dishes and drinks. People grow this herb on their kitchen window sill and add a few leaves to their early-morning brew! Stevia can enhance glucose tolerance and has no known adverse effects on blood glucose. This makes it an ideal dietary sugar supplement for patients with insulin resistance like those with polycystic ovarian disease and diabetics. Stevia can reduce mild elevations in blood pressure. So patients just beginning to show signs of hypertension may benefit from switching to stevia. Though better purified versions of stevia are now available in the market, some people still complain that it is cloyingly sweet and has a bitter aftertaste

Monk Fruit or Lo Han Guo is an ancient Chinese fruit about 300 times sweeter than sugar. The ancient Chinese used it for medicinal purposes in treating obesity, diabetes, and cancer because it is rich in antioxidants and anti-inflammatory substances. The Chinese also use it as a dietary sugar supplement. Nectresse, made by Splenda, has a combination of monk fruit powder, erythritol, sugar, and molasses.

Pure Glucose (Dextrose) does not contain any fructose and is a safer dietary sugar supplement. Since it is only 70 per cent as sweet as table sugar, more of it has to be used to sweeten a food product. This makes it a more expensive supplement.

GLYCEMIC INDEX OF SWEETENERS

Glucose 100
High Fructose Corn Syrup 100
White Sugar 68
Honey 62
Blackstrap Molasses 55
Maple Syrup 54
Agave Nectar 15
Xylitol 7

Since *any* sweetener can decrease insulin sensitivity it is always best to steer clear of *all* of them if the patient has diabetes, insulin resistance, dyslipidemia, hypertension, or is struggling with weight issues. A diabetic can manage without sugar and sugar substitutes by using a teaspoon of chopped dates or raisins or figs to sweeten a breakfast bowl of oatmeal or porridge or sheera. A sprinkling of cinnamon powder or vanilla extract will also enhance the taste and provide health benefits. Skip diet beverages in favour of buttermilk and unsweetened nimbu pani. If this is not possible, then it is best to regularly monitor post-meal blood sugars and identify which sweetener causes the least spike in blood glucose levels.

6

Controlling Diabetes with Herbs, Spices, and Supplements

Herbs and spices play a major role in our life. They enhance the pleasure that we derive from food and play a crucial role in shaping cuisine and adding interest to food. An aromatic meal, simple though it may be, will always be remembered. A pinch of paprika, a few strands of saffron, a dash of pepper powder, a teaspoon of lemon zest—all offer an opportunity to add flavour to food without the need of unhealthy excess salt, sugar, and fat. Herbs and spices are invaluable in folk medicine as well as in Chinese, Ayurvedic, herbal, and naturopathic treatments. Ancient Egyptians used various spices to enliven daily meals; they used the resinous pot herb myrrh in cosmetics, toothpaste, and lotions and they even used cinnamon and the bark of the cassia tree (Chinese cinnamon) to embalm the dead!

Although they are often used together, herbs and spices are not one and the same thing. Herbs are the aromatic leaves of plants like basil, bay leaf, chives, coriander, dill, fennel, mint, etc. They can be used in a variety of forms: fresh, mulled, dried, finely chopped, crushed, or even steeped in hot water. Since high heat can spoil their flavour, herbs should be added towards the end of the cooking process, when the food temperature is not very high. Spices like cardamom, cinnamon, paprika, cloves, fenugreek seeds, ginger, pepper, and nutmeg have a stronger flavour than herbs. They are obtained from the roots, seeds, berries, buds, flowers, fruits, and even the barks of the plant or tree. Spices are added at the start of the cooking process.

As a practitioner of naturopathy, I strongly believe that the humble spice box found in most kitchens is a source of help for diabetic patients. Coupled with some basic herbs, they can go a long way in aiding a diabetic in keeping a tight control over his blood glucose level. When blood glucose levels are high, protein glycation occurs. This in turn produces compounds that promote inflammation in the cells. These are known as AGE compounds (advanced glycation end products). Researchers have found a strong link between the polyphenol content in herbs and spices and their ability to block the formation of these AGE compounds.

Most of our commonly used dried herbs and spices can help block the inflammation that can keep diabetes and other chronic diseases uncontrolled. The inflammation-inhibiting antioxidant compounds called polyphenols found in cloves and cinnamon can help lower blood glucose as well as blood cholesterol values. Thus, the onset of many of the diabetes-linked complications like coronary heart disease, nephropathy, neuropathy, and retinopathy can be delayed or even be prevented from occurring. Fenugreek seeds and fenugreek leaves, *Gymnema sylvestre* or gudmar, sage, tarragon, curry leaves, rosemary, dill, turmeric, oregano, ginger, garlic, sesame seeds, and marjoram have a similar, albeit weaker, action.

However, be warned that indiscriminate self-supplementation can cause more serious harm than good. For example, the leaves of the gudmar plant (*Gymnema sylvestre*) are beneficial in lowering blood glucose levels. If a diabetic patient also has hypothyroidism, then the use of gudmar will have the opposite effect. The blood glucose level will rise. Hence it is best that you consult a knowledgeable healthcare practitioner who will work out the herb and spice combination best suited for your condition. Be sure to list out and discuss all your health issues and the daily supplements and medications you are taking. This will help your healthcare practioner assess your condition with ease and put you on the road to recovery as quickly as possible. At no time should you decrease or stop allopathic medication, unless your diabetologist deems it fit.

Here is a description of some of the herbs, spices, and supplements—listed in alphabetical order—related to diabetes and blood glucose control. Do consult your naturopath or healthcare practitioner before taking them or combining them yourself.

Astragalus: is a perennial native to China and Korea. Its root powder helps NIDDM patients control their blood glucose levels. It is an adaptogen, so if the blood glucose levels are high, it helps lower them. Conversely, if the blood glucose levels are low and the patient is experiencing symptoms of hypoglycemia, astragalus root powder helps to increase the blood glucose levels. In other words, it really helps to balance and keep the blood glucose levels as near to normal as possible. Astragalus root powder or extract improves the transport of glucose in muscle tissue. Excess blood glucose binds to cells and forms complexes called advanced glycation end products (AGEs) in a process known as protein glycation. This causes cellular inflammation, oxidation, and an increased pace of cellular aging. Astragalus root powder prevents this from happening. It is best to start with a 5 gm dosage per day and then gradually increase to 15 gm. Very high doses suppress the immune system which can be harmful for diabetics on immune-suppressing drugs. So diabetics with autoimmune diseases like rheumatoid arthritis, multiple sclerosis, Hashimotos thyroiditis, lupus, and Graves' disease should not take this extract. It is also best avoided by pregnant and lactating diabetic women.

Alpha-Linolenic Acid (ALA): is an antioxidant that protects against cell damage. ALA is currently being studied to find out if it can help with NIDDM, because of its role in reducing diabetic neuropathy. Supplements of ALA reduce symptoms like pain, tingling, and prickling in the feet, legs, and hands generally caused by nerve damage in the feet, legs or hands. ALA improves insulin sensitivity and lowers the rate of kidney damage. Several studies have found that ALA can improve insulin resistance. It may also help protect the retina from some of the damage that occurs in diabetic retinopathy. Foods like red meat, liver, kidney, yeast, rice bran, yam, potato, beets, carrot, tomato, dark green leafy vegetables like spinach, fenugreek, Brussels sprouts and broccoli, contain ALA in small amounts. Since ALA can lower blood glucose, diabetics taking medication should consult their diabetologist before starting on ALA supplements because it can cause hypoglycemia.

Allspice: is also known as pimento or Jamaican pepper. The British gave this West Indian tree with berry-like fruit its name because they couldn't decide which spice it was! Allspice has flavours of cinnamon, nutmeg, and cloves. It has been traditionally used as a digestion stimulant to cure flatulence. It is also used to treat rheumatism and arthritis as it is anti-inflammatory and soothes the joints and muscles. Allspice is also used to treat stomach ache, vomiting, diarrohea, and fever. Women can use it to soothe menstrual cramps. It is also used to help with blood glucose control. Make an allspice tea by steeping for 10 minutes a teaspoon of whole allspice along with 10 fenugreek seeds in 250 ml hot water. Have this thrice a day, after each meal. However, cancer patients, pregnant women, and women who are breastfeeding should avoid this.

Basil: is a member of the mint family. There are many types of basil which differ in taste and aroma. Holy basil, or tulsi, is an important plant used in Ayurvedic medicine. The leaves of the holy basil plant contain essential oils like eugenol. Research on NIDDM patients shows that holy basil leaves may improve the function of the beta cells of the islets of Langerhans of the pancreas. This improvement helps to increase the secretion of insulin, thereby preventing major fluctuation in both fasting as well as post-meal blood glucose levels. Holy basil is a powerful antioxidant. Chew on 5 tulsi leaves every morning, followed by a shot of lemon juice, or have a mug of warm tulsi lemon tea after carbohydrate-rich meals.

Bergamot: is a citrus plant grown in Calabria, Italy which gives Earl Grey tea its unmistakable and unique flavour, making it a favourite among tea lovers worldwide. Bergamot extract helps to improve the lipid profile by reducing triglycerides, LDL cholesterol, as well as the total blood cholesterol levels. It also helps increase HDL levels. It reduces blood glucose levels by suppressing the synthesis of glucose in the liver. Currently, this extract is being researched as an alternative to statin drugs.

Bitter Melon (karela): contains three substances with anti-diabetic properties, namely charantin, vicine, and an insulin-like compound called polypeptide-p. These substances help reduce blood glucose levels. Bitter melon also suppresses the appetite. Bitter melon is rich in vitamins A, B1, B2, and C. It also has iron. It helps prevent the complications associated with diabetes. Bitter melon juice should be drunk in the morning on an empty stomach.

Cassia bark: or Chinese cinnamon is sweeter-tasting than cinnamon. Chinese herbalists have been using it for centuries to increase insulin sensitivity and control blood glucose levels in Type 2 diabetics. Since it has coumarin, an anti-coagulant, it should not be taken regularly and in large amounts by diabetics with cardiovascular disease who are on blood thinners. Cinnamon contains very little natural coumarin.

Infuse a 2-inch piece of cassia bark, 2 strands of saffron, and 1 teaspoon grated ginger in 200 ml hot water. Drink this immediately after lunch and dinner. Add a sachet of green tea to this brew for added health benefits.

Chamomile: is a great relaxer well known for calming the mind, body, and soul. Chamomile tea helps with headaches and migraines, irritability, mood swings, insomnia, menstrual cramps, and the hot flushes associated with menopause. It is also good for soothing sensitive skin. Chamomile tea has post-meal blood glucose-lowering effects and also protects the beta cells of the islets of Langerhans of the pancreas from the harmful effects of hyperglycemia and oxidative stress. Since chamomile contains the anti-coagulant coumarin, it should be avoided by patients with bleeding disorders and those on blood-thinning medication. It should also be avoided during pregnancy because it acts as a uterine stimulant and increases the chance of a miscarriage.

Chia seeds: is a 'superfood' used by Aztec warriors and runners, who sustained themselves for an entire day on just one tablespoon of the seeds. Chia helps to build muscles and tissues. Chia forms a barrier between carbohydrates and enzymes, slowing down the production of glucose from carbohydrate-rich food. Chia also decreases the speed at which glucose enters the bloodstream, which obviously helps diabetics tremendously. These tiny seeds pack a big nutritional punch. Chia seeds are an excellent source of healthy Omega-3 fatty acids (Alpha-Linolenic acid), antioxidants, proteins, vitamins, minerals like calcium, manganese, and phosphorus, and soluble as well as insoluble dietary fibre. The fibre in chia seeds has a higher viscosity than the dietary fibers in beta-glucan and guar gum. Thus chia helps lower blood pressure and cholesterol too. Since it is tasteless, it can be added to a wide variety of foods. Just sprinkle some on your bowl of breakfast cereal, upma, poha, dalia, lapsi, toast, or even salads and raitas, or blend it into lassi, buttermilk, smoothies, fruit and vegetable juices. When soaked in water it forms a chia gel which makes an excellent ingredient in jams, puddings, and baked goods. Chia seeds are different from sabjia seeds, which they are often confused with. They do not reduce serum estrogen levels like sabjia seeds.

Chromium: is an essential mineral present in small amounts in egg yolk, coffee, nuts, broccoli, green beans, meat, shellfish, corn oil, Brewer's yeast, whole grain, and high-bran breakfast cereals. Since it is present in a wide variety of foods, a deficiency state is not very common. However, when food is processed, its chromium content decreases. Chromium may improve insulin function because it is an essential co-factor in the action of insulin. Chromium reduces both fasting as well as post-meal blood glucose levels. It also reduces the symptoms of diabetes like frequent urination, fatigue, and thirst. Gestational diabetics can manage their diabetes better with chromium. Chromium is safe in low doses, but may cause a drop in blood sugar or kidney problems if overused.

Cinnamon: is a well-known spice and has been used in traditional Chinese medicine for thousands of years. As a strong antioxidant, antimicrobial agent, and fat burner, it has been used to treat a variety of ailments such as headaches, toothache, bad breath, loss of appetite, dyspepsia, the common cold, inflammation, wounds, nausea, vomiting, flatulence, and diarrhoea. Cinnamon also reduces blood glucose, triglyceride, and total cholesterol and LDL cholesterol levels in NIDDM patients. The inclusion of cinnamon in the diet of people with Type 2 diabetes reduces risk factors associated with diabetes and cardiovascular diseases.

Simmer a 2-inch stick of cinnamon with 5 green cardamoms, 2 cloves, and a 1-inch slice of ginger in 300 ml water for 10 minutes. Steep this overnight. In the morning heat this decoction, strain, and drink warm on an empty stomach. Cinnamon can be added to oat porridge, smoothies, soups, stews, curries, chutneys, baked dishes, stewed fruit, tea, and coffee.

Cloves: are a magic spice. They have powerful germicidal properties and are used in dental care for relieving toothache, sore gums, and oral ulcers. Clove oil relaxes the mind and reduces mental exhaustion, depression, anxiety, memory loss, insomnia, and fatigue. Chewing on a clove helps relieve the discomfort of peptic ulcers as well as stomach-related conditions like nausea, hiccups, motion sickness, and vomiting. Cloves purify the blood and help in stabilizing blood glucose levels. Known for their hot, spicy, pungent flavour, cloves are a favourite seasoning spice for meats, baked goods, and beverages.

Curry leaves: are a common seasoning in Indian dishes, especially those from south India. They contain minerals like iron, calcium, copper, phosphorus, magnesium, and vitamins A, B, C, and E. They are also a source of antioxidants. Due to their mineral content, curry leaves help activate the beta cells of the islets of Langerhans of the pancreas, helping to control blood glucose levels in Type 2 diabetics. Curry leaves may help in the production of alpha-amylase, an enzyme produced in the pancreas, which helps to break down starch from the carbohydrates in a meal. Hence they help to decrease the rate of starch-to-glucose breakdown and prevent too much glucose from entering the bloodstream. The antioxidants in curry leaves prevent cellular damage. Tempering food with curry leaves helps incorporate it into the daily diet. But remember to eat the leaves rather than push them to the side of the plate! Curry leaf chutneys can also be made a part of the daily diet. Else just chew on 10 leaves every morning.

Flaxseed: are brown seeds which look like flattened apple seeds and contain protein, lignan fibre, and, most importantly, high levels of the essential Omega-3 fatty acid called Alpha-Linolenic acid (ALA). They are a low-glycemic index food and they help to stabilize blood glucose levels and prevent spikes. The phytoestrogen lignans in flaxseed slows down the rate of absorption of glucose through the small intestine, thus helping to lower blood glucose levels. A Type 2 diabetic can bring down his HbA1c levels if he takes a tablespoon of flaxseed daily. Sprinkle freshly ground flaxseed along with cinnamon powder on toast, porridge, or breakfast cereals, blend it into smoothies, or use it in chutneys and spreads.

Fenugreek: are bitter seeds as well as leaves that protect the liver, lower triglycerides and blood glucose levels, improve the lipid profile, and act as cleansing agents. Galactomannan, the dietary fibre present in fenugreek seeds, decreases the rate at which carbohydrate digestion takes place, stimulates insulin secretion in the pancreas, and lowers the glucose absorption.

Soak a teaspoon of fenugreek seeds in 100 ml water overnight and have this on rising. Remember to chew the seeds well.

Garlic: contains allicin, a sulphur-containing compound that gives it its antimicrobial, antibacterial, antifungal, and antioxidant properties. Garlic helps to increase the amount of insulin released by the pancreas, regulate blood glucose levels, and protect the heart from diabetes-induced cardiomyopathy. However, diabetics who are bleeders should avoid using garlic to lower their blood glucose levels. Allicin works best if the cloves of garlic are crushed or chopped and kept aside exposed to air for some time. Chew two of these cloves daily, preferably on an empty stomach. This will also help with hypertension and hypercholesterolemia. Alternatively, use freshly ground garlic paste in dips, chutneys, spreads, sauces, and gravies.

Ginger: in the raw root form, is an effective treatment for the complications associated with diabetes. It inhibits the effects of the enzyme alpha-glucosidase, increases insulin production, and decreases blood glucose levels. Thus it helps in long-term blood glucose control. Ginger improves cell sensitivity to insulin and reduces C-reactive protein, cholesterol and other lipid factions which lead to cardiac disease. It may also protect against kidney damage in diabetics with poor glucose control.

Add a couple of raw ginger slices to a litre or two of water and drink this through the day or use 1–2 teaspoon grated ginger in salads, raitas, etc. to see the health benefits.

Ginseng: is an adaptogenic herb which enhances general well-being. It can help control blood glucose levels possibly by boosting insulin production in Type 2 diabetics. Research on its long-term safety and effectiveness is still being conducted.

Gymnema sylvestre: are leaves that contain glucoside and compounds called gymnemic acids. These decrease the rate at which glucose is transported from the intestines to the bloodstream. Gymnema contains substances that decrease the absorption of sugar from the intestine. Gymnema may also increase the amount of insulin in the body and increase the cellular growth in the pancreas. Both Type 1 and Type 2 diabetics benefit from these leaves. They show reductions in blood glucose as well as in HbA1C levels. Research is being conducted to check the effects of gymnema on diabetics with hypothyroidism. So these patients should avoid using gymnema leaves.

Jamun: is one of the best fruits for diabetic patients. Its seed contains glycoside, jamboline, gallic acid, and essential oils. It has antioxidant and anti-inflammatory properties. Jamboline has the ability to control the excessive conversion of starch into sugar. It also helps in reducing the quantity of sugar in urine. A diabetic patient should have 1 teaspoon of this powder twice a day (morning and evening). Studies show that jamun may protect the pancreatic gland by restoring protective enzymes such as glutathione back to normal levels. 1 teaspoon of jamun seed powder should be taken in a glass of water twice a day.

Magnesium: is abundantly present in a wide variety of foods, e.g., nuts and seeds like flaxseed, melon seeds, pumpkin seeds, cocoa, and dark green leafy vegetables. A high-magnesium diet can lower the risk of developing Type 2 diabetes. A magnesium deficiency can arise if the diet is deficient in magnesium or if the kidney excretes large amounts of magnesium. If there is a magnesium deficiency then the person can develop insulin resistance, impaired glucose tolerance, and decreased levels of insulin secretion. Magnesium improves insulin sensitivity thus lowering insulin resistance. Magnesium and insulin work together. Without magnesium, the pancreas is not able to secrete enough insulin to control blood glucose levels. Supplementation with 200–500 mg may be required.

Turmeric: a relative of ginger, has a compound called curcumin which gives turmeric its orangish-yellow colour. It helps to decrease blood glucose as well as blood cholesterol levels. It should not be used by diabetics on anti-platelet and anti-coagulant medications. The antioxidant and anti-inflammatory agents of curcumin help to fight the disease and strengthen the immune system of the body. Turmeric can also be consumed daily to prevent diabetes. Mix half a teaspoon of turmeric powder with 2 teaspoons of lemon juice and 5 crushed basil leaves. Add to 2 tablespoons of yoghurt and eat after lunch and dinner.

7

Healthy Recipes

STUFFED ZUCCHINI
Serves 4

Ingredients

 4 medium-sized zucchini
 1 red bell pepper, deseeded and chopped into small squares
 1 green bell pepper, deseeded and chopped into small squares
 2 medium-sized tomatoes, peeled, deseeded and chopped
 2 spring onions, finely chopped
 2 teaspoons garlic, finely chopped
 2 stalks celery, finely chopped
 2 tablespoons coriander, finely chopped
 1 tablespoon pumpkin seeds
 4 tablespoons hung curd
 1 tablespoon olive oil
 Salt and pepper to taste

Trim the ends of the zucchini without peeling it. Lightly cook it in a large pan of salted water and drain out the water.

Cut the lightly cooked zucchini lengthwise in halves and scoop out the flesh using a scooper or a teaspoon. Tightly wrap these zucchini shells in cling film and refrigerate till needed.

Blend the olive oil and hung curd well, and add salt and pepper to taste. Then add the bell peppers, tomatoes, spring onions, garlic, celery, coriander, and pumpkin seeds. Mix well. Refrigerate.

When ready to serve, remove from the refrigerator and spoon this filling into the zucchini shells.

Nutrient Value: Energy: 143 kcals; Protein: 7 g; Carbs: 8 g; Fat: 9 g; Fibre: 6 g; Sugar: 1 g; Salt: 0.94 g

Marinated Baked Tofu
Serves 4

Ingredients

400 gm extra-firm tofu (can be substituted with low-fat paneer)
1 tablespoon garlic, finely chopped
1 tablespoon ginger, finely chopped
1 tablespoon rice vinegar
1 tablespoon sesame oil
2 teaspoons green chilli paste
4 tablespoons soy sauce
1 teaspoon olive oil

Firmly press down the block of tofu (or paneer) to remove any excess water. Chop into cubes.

Mix the ginger, garlic, chilli paste, soy sauce, rice vinegar, and sesame oil.

Pour this marinade over the tofu and refrigerate overnight.

Grease a non-stick baking tray with a teaspoon olive oil. Arrange the marinated tofu cubes on this and bake in a pre-heated oven at 160 °C till golden brown.

Nutrient Value: Energy: 224 kcals; Protein: 14 g; Carbs: 6 g; Fat: 16 g; Fibre: 5 g; Sugar: 2 g; Salt: 1.2 g

Spinach and Mixed-Grain Idlis
Serves 6

Ingredients

For the mixed-grain idli batter:
2 tablespoons rice, coarsely ground
2 tablespoons nachni atta
2 tablespoons oatmeal
1 tablespoon makai atta (coarsely ground cornmeal)
½ cup dahi
1 cup water
Salt to taste

For the spinach mixed-grain idlis:
150 gm mixed-grain idli batter
2 cups spinach leaves
2 green chillies

1 teaspoon oil
⅛ teaspoon mustard seeds
1 teaspoon channa dal
8–10 curry leaves
Salt to taste

Whisk the dahi with the water and add the other dry ingredients to make the mixed-grain idli batter. Leave overnight to ferment.

Temper the mustard seeds, channa dal, and curry leaves in 1 teaspoon oil.

Purée the spinach leaves along with the green chillies.

Take 1 cup of the mixed-grain idli batter and add the tempered mustard seeds, channa dal, curry leaves, and spinach chilli purée to it.

Add salt to taste.

Pour this batter into greased idli moulds and steam for 8 minutes.

Serve hot either plain or with green chutney or dahi.

Nutrient Value: Energy: 260 kcals; Protein: 6.5 g; Carbs: 45 g; Fat: 6 g; Fibre 7 g; Sugar: 2.2 g; Salt 0.87 g

Celery, Garlic, and Lentil Soup
Serves 6

Ingredients

150 gm red masoor dal, washed, soaked in water for 1 hour and drained
2 tablespoons finely chopped garlic
2 medium-sized onions, finely chopped

100 gm white pumpkin, finely chopped
1 tablespoon olive oil
2 tejpatta
2 stalks celery, finely chopped
1 teaspoon paprika
1 teaspoon oregano
Salt and pepper to taste
2 cups of water

Put all the ingredients, with the exception of the tejpatta and the olive oil, into the pressure cooker and cook for 20 minutes after the first whistle.

Temper the tejpatta in the olive oil.

Once the pressure cooker has cooled, open and stir the contents.

Adjust the consistency as well as the seasoning.

Purée the soup or leave as is.

Add the tempered tejpatta and simmer for 10 minutes.

Serve hot.

Nutrient Value: Energy: 190 kcals; Protein: 13 g; Carbs: 18 g; Fat: 7.5 g; Fibre: 2 g; Sugar: 1.4 g; Salt: 1.1 g

Mustard Chicken
Serves 6

Ingredients

1 kg boneless chicken, cut into medium-sized pieces
½ kg onions, finely chopped
4 green chillies, slit lengthwise

4 tablespoons yellow mustard paste or kasundi
Salt to taste
1 tablespoon olive oil

Sauté onions in 1 tablespoon olive oil, then add the slit green chillies and mustard paste.

Add chicken pieces and salt and cook till done, adding water if necessary.

When the chicken is cooked, remove the pieces and keep aside.

Reduce the remaining gravy till it acquires a sauce-like consistency.

Pour this sauce over the cooked chicken pieces
Serve warm.

Nutrient Value: Energy: 250 kcals; Protein: 28 g; Carbs: 12 g; Fat: 10 g; Fibre: 2 g; Sugar: 1.4 g; Salt: 1.53 g

BAKED POMFRET WITH MINT-AND-BASIL CHUTNEY
Serves 4

Ingredients

1 kg whole pomfret, scaled and cleaned
2 teaspoons coriander seeds, coarsely crushed
2 tablespoons grated ginger
1 tablespoon finely chopped garlic
3 tablespoons olive oil
2 lemons, deseeded and sliced
10 spring onions, halved
10 cherry tomatoes
10 peppercorns, crushed
Salt to taste

For the mint-and-basil chutney
2 tablespoons mint paste
2 tablespoons fresh basil paste
1 tablespoon lemon juice
1 tablespoon green chilli paste
1 tablespoon garlic paste
Salt to taste

Slash the pomfret diagonally on both sides and rub with grated ginger, chopped garlic, coarsely crushed coriander seeds, salt, and 1 tablespoon olive oil. Set aside for 20 minutes.

In a baking pan, place the cherry tomatoes, spring onion halves, lemon slices, crushed peppercorns, and the remaining 2 tablespoons of olive oil.

Place the pomfret on top of this and bake until the pomfret is cooked.

In the meantime, make the mint-and-basil chutney by simply mixing all the ingredients together.

Serve this chutney with the baked pomfret.

Nutrient Value: Energy: 269 kcals; Protein: 29 g; Carbs: 22 g; Fat: 7.3 g; Fibre: 3.1 g; Sugar: 1.6 g; Salt: 1.68 g

RED PEPPER AND PINE NUT RISOTTO
Serves 4

Ingredients

2 large red bell peppers
2 tablespoons yellow corn, boiled
1 tablespoon garlic, finely chopped

2 large tomatoes, deseeded and chopped
2 tejpatta
1 tablespoon olive oil
6 cups vegetable broth
2 cups Arborio rice (or brown rice), washed and drained
Salt and pepper to taste
1 tablespoon toasted pine nuts
6–8 basil leaves, chopped

Grill the red peppers, turning them often, until their skins are blistered. Remove from the grill and cover the peppers with a damp kitchen towel. Leave aside for 10 minutes. The skins will now come off very easily.

Remove the core and the seeds and slice the peppers.

Heat the oil and add tejpatta, chopped garlic, and chopped tomatoes. Allow to cook for some time and then add the red bell pepper slices and the boiled corn.

Heat the vegetable broth in another pan. Add rice to the vegetable mixture and cook for 2–3 minutes.

Now add 2–3 cooking spoonfuls of the hot vegetable broth. Cook till the broth has been absorbed.

Continue adding the vegetable broth 2–3 cooking spoonfuls at a time, ensuring that the broth has been completely absorbed each time.

Season with salt and pepper once the rice is cooked (it should have a creamy consistency).

Remove from heat, cover, and keep aside for 10 minutes.

Before serving, add the toasted pine nuts and the chopped basil leaves.

Serve warm.

Nutrient Value: Energy: 234 kcals; Protein: 16 g; Carbs: 24 g; Fat: 8 g; Fibre: 3.8 g; Sugar: 1.7 g; Salt: 1.3 g

MILLET, SOY, AND BEAN SPROUT PARATHAS
Serves 6

Ingredients

- 200 gm soy granules, boiled
- 100 gm bean sprouts, steamed
- 300 gm millet (bajra) flour
- 100 gm wholewheat flour
- 1 teaspoon cumin seeds
- 1 green chilli, finely chopped
- 1 tablespoon ghee
- 1 tablespoon olive oil
- Salt to taste

Heat the olive oil in a pan; temper the cumin seeds and the green chilli. Add the soy granules and bean sprouts. Season with salt and cook for some time. Leave the mixture aside to cool.

Make a semi-soft dough with the millet and wholewheat flours, ½ tablespoon ghee, water, and salt.

Make small chappatis with this dough, stuff with the bean sprout and soy mixture, and seal and cook on a non-stick griddle, using the remaining ½ tablespoon ghee, till brown and crisp.

Serve hot with flaxseed chutney or a hung curd dip.

Nutrient Value: Energy: 248 kcals; Protein: 15 g; Carbs: 27 g; Fat: 9 g; Fibre: 3.7 g; Sugar: 1.6 g; Salt: 0.75 g

DALIA AND GREEN MOONG PULAO
Serves 4

Ingredients

- 100 gm dalia
- 100 gm green moong dal
- 2 tablespoons green coriander paste
- 2 medium-sized onions, chopped
- ½ teaspoon haldi powder
- 2 teaspoons ginger, grated
- 1 teaspoon cumin seeds
- 1 teaspoon garam masala powder
- 1 tablespoon sesame oil
- Salt to taste
- 2 cups hot water
- 2 tablespoons mint, finely chopped
- 2 tablespoons parsley, finely chopped
- 1 lemon

Wash and soak the green moong dal in cold water for 1 hour. Drain.

Wash and soak the dalia in hot water for 30 minutes. Drain.

In a pressure cooker, heat 1 tablespoon sesame oil and temper the cumin seeds. Then sauté the chopped onions and when they soften, add the dalia, green moong dal, grated ginger, coriander paste, haldi powder, and garam masala powder.

Add 2 cups hot water and salt to taste.

Pressure-cook for 1 whistle.

When ready to serve, stir in the chopped mint and parsley. Add the juice of 1 lemon and serve warm.

Nutrient Value: Energy: 256 kcals ; Protein: 22 g; Carbs: 26 g; Fat: 7 g; Fibre: 3.3 g; Sugar: 1.34 g; Salt: 1.2 g

MIXED-SEED AUBERGINE
Serves 4

Ingredients

- 1 large aubergine
- 2 tablespoons apple cider vinegar
- 1 tablespoon soy sauce
- 1 teaspoon dried ginger powder
- 1 teaspoon jaggery sugar
- 1 tablespoon sunflower oil
- 1 teaspoon sesame seeds, toasted
- 2 teaspoons pumpkin seeds, toasted
- 1 teaspoon melon seeds, toasted
- 1 teaspoon poppy seeds, toasted
- Juice of 1 lemon
- 1 tablespoon fresh coriander, chopped
- Salt to taste

Cut the aubergine into medium-sized pieces.

Mix the apple cider vinegar, soy sauce, ginger powder, salt, and jaggery sugar well and marinate the aubergine pieces in this for 1 hour.

Heat oil in a pan and sauté the marinated aubergine pieces.

Add some water, adjust the seasoning, and cook till tender.

Garnish with the mixed toasted seeds and the chopped coriander.

Add lemon juice just before serving.

Nutrient Value: Energy: 187 kcals; Protein: 12 g; Carbs: 10 g; Fat: 11 g; Fibre: 1.6 g; Sugar: 1.01 g; Salt: 0.88 g

OAT PANCAKES WITH VEGETABLE FILLING
Serves 4

Ingredients

For the pancakes
100 gm oat flour
50 gm wholewheat flour
1 egg
300 ml thin buttermilk
Salt to taste

For the filling
100 gm cabbage, finely chopped or shredded
50 gm French beans, finely chopped
50 gm carrots, diced
100 gm broccoli, chopped
4 button mushrooms, quartered
1 tablespoon sesame oil
1 teaspoon onion seeds
1 teaspoon grated ginger
1 teaspoon paprika
Salt to taste

In a mixing bowl, mix the oat and wholewheat flours.

Make a well in the centre, add the egg, salt, and buttermilk and mix well to make a smooth batter.

Lightly oil a heated non-stick griddle.

Pour enough batter to coat the base of the griddle while moving the griddle around.

Cook the pancake till the lower side no longer sticks to the griddle.

Flip it over and cook the other side.

Cook the remaining pancakes in the same way.

Heat 1 tablespoon sesame oil in a pan, add the onion seeds and grated ginger.

Toss in the vegetables and stir-fry until just crisp-tender.

Add the paprika and adjust the seasoning.

Stuff each pancake with this vegetable filling, roll up, and serve.

Nutrient Value: Energy: 260 kcals; Protein: 21 g; Carbs: 26 g; Fat: 8 g; Fibre: 3.5 g; Sugar: 1.7 g; Salt: 1.23 g

SPINACH, MINT, AND BUTTERMILK SOUP
Serves 4

Ingredients

200 gm spinach, blanched and puréed
2 tablespoons mint paste
500 ml vegetable stock
1 large onion, finely chopped
1 tablespoon finely chopped garlic
50 gm oat flour
200 ml thin buttermilk
1 teaspoon grated nutmeg
1 tablespoon vegetable oil
Salt and pepper to taste

Heat the vegetable oil in a pan and sauté the onion and garlic till it softens. Add the spinach purée, mint paste, and vegetable stock and bring to a boil.

Cook for 10 minutes.

Mix the oat flour with some water and add to the pan along with the nutmeg, salt, and pepper.

Cook till the soup thickens.

Cool slightly and then stir in the buttermilk.

Serve immediately.

Nutrient Value: Energy: 210 kcals; Protein: 21 g; Carbs: 18 g; Fat: 6 g; Fibre: 2.4 g; Sugar: 1.2 g; Salt: 1.1 g

DILL AND CUCUMBER SALAD
Serves 4

Ingredients

6 medium-sized cucumbers, peeled and diced
2 tablespoons dill, chopped
1 large onion, chopped
4 tablespoons hung curd
2 tablespoons balsamic vinegar
Salt to taste

In a mixing bowl, combine the hung curd, balsamic vinegar, chopped dill, and salt.

Add the chopped onions and cucumbers and stir gently so that the dressing lightly coats the onions and cucumbers.

Refrigerate for 20–30 minutes.

Serve cold.

Nutrient Value: Energy: 96 kcals; Protein: 7 g; Carbs: 8 g; Fat: 4 g; Fibre: 3.6 g; Sugar: 1 g; Salt: 0.79 g

DOODHI, OATMEAL, AND QUINOA THEPLAS
Serves 4

Ingredients

150 gm doodhi, grated
100 gm oat flour
100 gm quinoa flour
4 tablespoons wholewheat flour
1 tablespoon coriander, finely chopped
1 tablespoon mint, finely chopped
A pinch of heeng
1 teaspoon chopped green chilli
1 teaspoon ginger paste
Salt to taste
1 tablespoon peanut oil

Add some salt to the grated doodhi, leave aside for 5 minutes, then squeeze out the excess water.

Add the remaining ingredients with the exception of the oil and make a soft dough.

Divide the dough into equal-sized balls and roll out medium-sized theplas.

Cook the theplas on a non-stick griddle.

Serve hot.

Nutrient Value: Energy: 242 kcals; Protein: 19 g; Carbs: 23.5 g; Fat: 8 g; Fibre: 3.5 g; Sugar: 1.6 g; Salt: 0.89 g

Peach and Vanilla Bean Shake
Serves 1

Ingredients

    100 ml soy or skim milk
    100 gm low-fat yoghurt
    1 peach, chopped
    1 vanilla bean, slit lengthwise and extracted
    Stevia sugar substitute to taste
    1 cup ice cubes

In a blender, combine all the ingredients with the exception of the ice cubes. Blend till smooth and bubbly.

Add the ice cubes and blend again.

Pour into a tall glass and serve immediately.

Nutrient Value: Energy: 231 kcals; Protein: 14.6 g; Carbs: 18.5 g; Fat: 11 g; Fibre: 2.2 g; Sugar: 1.67 g; Salt: 0.87 g

Antioxidant Booster Juice
Serves 1

Ingredients

    1 green apple, deseeded, cored, and cut into pieces
    20 spinach leaves
    20 parsley leaves
    2 stalks celery
    2 tomatoes, peeled and deseeded
    2 tablespoons aloe juice
    ½ teaspoon fenugreek seed powder

1 tablespoon lemon juice
1 cup cold water

Place all the ingredients in a blender and blend well.
Serve immediately.

Nutrient Value: Energy: 106 kcals; Protein: 2.5 g; Carbs: 19.5 g; Fat: 2 g; Fibre: 5.1 g; Sugar: 2.4 g; Salt: 1.67 g

BAKED BROWN RICE PUDDING
Serves 4

Ingredients

200 gm brown rice
500 ml skim milk
300 ml water
1 teaspoon cinnamon powder
½ teaspoon grated nutmeg
¼ teaspoon salt
2 eggs, whisked
1 tablespoon vanilla essence
Stevia sugar substitute to taste

Wash and soak the brown rice in water for an hour, then drain.
Boil the water and add ½ teaspoon cinnamon powder and salt.
When the water begins to boil, add the brown rice and cook until most of the water is absorbed. Then add the milk, whisked eggs, vanilla essence, and stevia and let it simmer for 5 minutes.

Pour this warm rice mixture into a greased baking dish or small ramekin moulds.

Bake in a preheated oven at 180 °C for 30–40 minutes.

Dust with the remaining ½ teaspoon cinnamon powder and serve warm or chilled.

Nutrient Value: Energy: 265 kcals; Protein: 20 g; Carbs: 26 g; Fat: 9 g; Fibre: 3.7 g; Sugar: 2.6 g; Salt: 1.33 g

Baked Apples
Serves 2

Ingredients

- 2 medium-sized apples
- 1 tablespoon pumpkin seeds
- 1 tablespoon chironji
- 2 teaspoons sesame seeds
- 2 teaspoons poppyseed
- 1 tablespoon dessicated coconut
- 2 dried apricots, soaked overnight and chopped
- 8 black raisins, deseeded and chopped
- 2 teaspoons cinnamon powder
- 4 tablespoons lemon juice
- 1 tablespoon vegetable oil

Core the apples without chopping them.

Heat the oil in a pan and add the pumpkin seeds, chironji, sesame seeds, poppyseed, and dessicated coconut. Heat until light brown and turn off the heat.

Add the chopped apricots and black raisins.

Lastly, add the lemon juice and cinnamon powder.

Divide this mixture into two and stuff each cored apple with it.

Wrap each apple in aluminium foil and bake in a preheated oven at 150 °C for 20–30 minutes until the apples soften.

Serve warm.

Nutrient Value: Energy: 197 kcals; Protein: 12 g; Carbs: 19 g; Fat: 8 g; Fibre: 3.4 g; Sugar: 2.45 g; Salt: 1.7 g

Papaya Halwa
Serves 4

Ingredients

300 gm papaya, grated
2 tablespoons skim milk powder
1 teaspoon cardamom powder
1 tablespoon ghee
1 teaspoon chironji, roasted
Stevia sugar substitute if needed to sweeten

Heat ghee in a pan and cook the grated papaya in it. Cook the fruit until the juice has evaporated.

Add the milk powder and cardamom powder and stir well.

Remove from the heat, cool, taste, and then add stevia if needed.

Garnish with roasted chironji.

Serve warm or cold.

Nutrient Value: Energy: 166 kcals; Protein: 7 g; Carbs: 23 g; Fat: 5 g; Fibre: 3 g; Sugar: 3.1 g; Salt: 0.38 g

FIG AND COFFEE ICE CREAM
Serves 4

Ingredients

4 dried figs
300 ml skim milk
2 tablespoons skim milk powder
1 teaspoon cornflour
4 slices brown bread, toasted and crumbed
Stevia sugar substitute to taste
2 teaspoons coffee powder

Soak the figs in water for an hour. Chop and keep aside.

Combine the skim milk powder, coffee powder, and cornflour with 2 tablespoons cold milk to make a smooth paste.

Bring the rest of the milk to boil and add this paste.

Stir and cook till the mixture thickens. Cool.

When the mixture has cooled, add the brown bread crumbs and the desired amount of stevia.

Pour the mixture into an aluminium pan, cover with a sheet of plastic and then with a firm lid. Freeze overnight.

Thaw the frozen mixture and whisk well.

Add the softened chopped figs and repeat the aluminium-pan process. The plastic sheet prevents the water of condensation from the lid, from forming icicles in the ice cream.

Freeze until it sets.

Nutrient Value: Energy: 265 kcals; Protein: 16 g; Carbs: 22 g; Fat: 12.5 g; Fibre: 4 g; Sugar: 3.68 g; Salt: 1.03 g

8

The Way Forward

BARIATRIC SURGERY

During recent years, it has become clear that the gastrointestinal tract constitutes the largest and most varied endocrine organ of the human body. More than forty different types of metabolic hormones originate from the gastrointestinal tract, and several of these hormones exert a considerable impact on glucose metabolism and appetite regulation. This in turn impacts body weight and blood glucose levels.

Faced with the diabetes epidemic, scientists have made advances in the treatment of a condition that was once thought of as irreversible. Bariatric surgery, from the Greek 'baros' meaning 'weight', is synonymous with weight-loss surgery. Bariatric surgery has been found to help more than 80 per cent of patients with Type 2 diabetes by resulting in acute glucose-lowering effects. The most common types of bariatric surgery are the Roux-en-Y Gastric Bypass (RYGB), Biliopancreatic Diversion Surgery, Sleeve Gastrectomy, and Gastric Banding.

Bariatric surgery is now being recommended to all people who have a BMI of 35 or more, whether they have diabetes or not. This is to help prevent them from developing diabetes in the future. Type 2 diabetics with a BMI greater than 30 are also opting for bariatric surgery when they have poorly controlled diabetes. In fact, in people with Type 2 diabetes, normal plasma glucose was restored within seven days of RYBG or Biliopancreatic Diversion Surgery, the reason for this being that the liver fat level is closely related to hepatic insulin sensitivity for control of blood glucose production. One form of bariatric surgery called Sleeve Gastrectomy resolved the diabetic state more effectively. Evidently, the body weight-lowering effect of these bariatric operations contributes to the long-term improvements in glucose metabolism. Shunting food directly to the lower intestine stimulates a substance called glucagon-like peptide 1 (GLP-1), which can increase the production of the hormone insulin.

Whether bariatric surgery by itself improves the patient's metabolic function due to modifications of gastrointestinal factors or purely because of the low-calorie intake in the first few months after surgery remains controversial.

Periodic Fasting

Researchers at the Intermountain Heart Institute, Intermountain Medical Center in Murray, Utah noticed that after ten to twelve hours of fasting, the body starts scavenging for other sources of energy throughout the body to sustain itself. The body pulls LDL cholesterol (bad cholesterol) from the fat cells and uses it as an energy source. Fasting can reduce cholesterol levels in pre-diabetic people over an extended period of time. This periodic fasting can help to combat one of the major diabetic risk factors. Routine water-only one-day fasting was associated with lower blood glucose levels and weight loss. However, this type of fasting should not be carried out more than twice a month, and that too not by insulin-dependent diabetics. If, at any time during the fasting, a diabetic on oral hypoglycemic feels dizzy because of a drop in blood glucose levels, he should immediately break his fast with some fruit.

BIONIC PANCREAS

Diabetics need to maintain a tight control over their blood glucose levels in order to enjoy good health for a long time and to delay or avoid the onset of various serious complications associated with the disease. IDDM patients have to check their blood glucose levels several times a day and after each check-up they have to inject a particular dosage of insulin which correlates with their blood glucose level. This insulin reaches them either through an injection or through a pocket-sized pump with a tube that goes under their skin. Even with the most sophisticated devices, it is not easy to prevent hypoglycemia and hyperglycemia. That diabetics have a malfunctioning pancreas which does not make sufficient insulin is a well-known fact. What is not so well known is the fact that their pancreas does not release glucagon, a hormone which raises blood glucose, whenever there is hypoglycemia.

Scientists from Boston University and Massachusetts General Hospital have come together to develop a 'bionic pancreas' to help patients with IDDM break free from the anxiety-filled daily ordeal of keeping a tight control over their blood glucose level. They are working together to make automated blood glucose control a reality in the near future. Engineers from Boston University have developed a wearable device that constantly monitors a patient's blood glucose. The device is a closed-loop bionic pancreas system that uses continuous glucose monitoring along with subcutaneous delivery of both rapid-acting insulin to lower blood glucose, and glucagon to raise blood glucose, as needed. Unlike previous artificial pancreases that could only correct high blood glucose by giving a particular dosage of insulin, this new device can also alter low blood glucose levels by giving glucagon in the prescribed amounts. In this way, the bionic pancreas mimics the activity of a normal, healthy pancreas. The bionic pancreas is mainly for patients with IDDM. It automatically records blood glucose levels every five minutes and then takes a decision about the dosage of insulin and glucagon. The bionic pancreas device comprises of a phone hardwired to a continuous glucose monitor and two pumps. One pump can deliver insulin in response to hyperglycemia. The other pump can deliver glucagon whenever there is hypoglycemia. Clinical trials are currently on and millions of diabetics the world over are eagerly awaiting the trial results.

The end goal is to find a complete cure for diabetes. As long as this goal remains elusive, the development of the 'bionic pancreas'—a drug-delivery device that responds to glucose concentrations—is the long-term goal of many scientists working to achieve greater success in diabetes therapy. This device has the ability to administer both insulin as well as glucagon as and when needed. Thus it can consistently keep diabetics happy, healthy, and safe from both hyperglycemia as well as hypoglycemia. Patients and their relatives are anxiously waiting to see what can be accomplished through the innovative and visionary efforts of the scientific and medical community.

THE FIBROBLAST GROWTH FACTOR 1 (FGF1) PROTEIN

Scientists from the Salk Institute for Biological Studies have published a paper in the journal *Nature* which could be termed as a breakthrough in diabetes treatment. The Salk scientists have shown that the endocrinization of the acidic FGF1 produces a potent insulin hormone sensitizer. Their experiments on mice with diet-induced diabetes have shown that a single injection of the acidic FGF1 protein found in pituitary extracts can keep the blood glucose levels within the normal range for two days or more. This diet-induced diabetes in mice is the equivalent of Type 2 diabetes in humans. When the mice were overfed, they developed diabetes and their liver tissues showed unhealthy cells filled with fat. Subsequent to regular treatment with FGF1 injections, the liver cells lost the fat and successfully absorbed sugar from the bloodstream. In time, the blood glucose levels stabilized and the cells began to resemble the normal cells of non-diabetic mice.

Excess weight and inactivity can lead to Type 2 diabetes. Glucose accumulates in the blood stream because of insufficient production of the hormone insulin by the beta cells of the islets of Langerhans in the pancreas. Sometimes blood cells become resistant to insulin and fail to absorb blood glucose. Since there is no cure for the disease, diabetes is a chronic condition which can cause serious health problems if not treated effectively. Successful management of this condition can be brought about by a combination of exercise, diet, and medication. The current lot of diabetic medications boosts insulin hormone levels and alters insulin resistance. Medications that stimulate the pancreas to produce more insulin can cause the blood glucose levels to fall drastically and lead to hypoglycemia which can be fatal. They can also cause other side effects.

The team from Salk found that the long-term treatment with FGF1 not only keeps the blood glucose levels normal but also reverses sensitivity to the hormone insulin. Most importantly, this new form of treatment does not cause hypoglycemia and many more side effects common to other forms of blood glucose control. FGF1 helps the body respond quickly to the hormone insulin. Even with a single dose, the blood glucose levels fell to near-normal levels in all the diabetic mice. When healthy mice were injected with FGF1, this lowering effect on blood glucose was not seen. Even high doses of FGF1 did not trigger hypoglycemia and other side effects in the diabetic mice. This is because FGF1 metabolizes very quickly in the body and targets only certain type of cells. Hence hypoglycemia does not result. Instead, the injections restored the body's natural ability to regulate the hormone insulin and the blood glucose levels.

The Salk scientists are now planning trials of FGF1 protein injections on humans and to then fine-tune this protein into a therapeutic diabetic medication. Millions of diabetics the world over will benefit if the perfect variation of this protein, that affects the blood glucose levels and not cell growth, is developed. Indeed, it will be a very effective tool for blood glucose control.

9

A Dictionary for Diabetics

A

Acanthosis nigricans: is a skin condition that results in the darkening and thickening of the skin around the nape of the neck, the elbow and knee creases, and also the armpit skin. It can be a warning sign of impaired glucose tolerance and insulin resistance. This skin condition is a warning sign for people who have pre-diabetes or NIDDM.

Acarbose: is an oral medicine used to treat Type 2 diabetes. As an alpha-glucosidase inhibitor, it blocks the enzymes that digest starches in food, resulting in a slower rise in blood glucose throughout the day. E.g., Precose.

ACE inhibitor: Angiotensin Converting Enzyme inhibitor is an oral medicine that lowers blood pressure. It widens the blood vessels in order to improve the amount of blood the heart pumps. For people with diabetes, especially those with proteinuria, it also helps slow down the rate of kidney damage. E.g., Minipril, Losapril, Amlo-B.

Acesulfame potassium: is a zero-calorie dietary sweetener and has no nutritional value. It aggravates low blood sugar attacks and is carcinogenic or cancer-causing.

Acetohexamide: is an oral medicine used to treat Type 2 diabetes. As a sulfonylurea, it helps the pancreas make more insulin and also helps the body make better use of this insulin, thereby lowering blood glucose. E.g., Dymelor.

Acute: describes something that happens suddenly and for a short time, e.g. acute stomach pain, acute renal failure.

Adhesive capsulitis: or frozen shoulder is a chronic condition of the shoulder that may also be associated with diabetes. It results in pain and loss of the ability to move the shoulder in all directions. Physiotherapy is needed to ease the pain and restore movement.

Adult-onset diabetes: is known as NIDDM or Type 2 diabetes. Younger people are also being diagnosed with this condition.

Albuminuria: is a condition in which the urine has more than normal amounts of a protein called albumin. It may indicate nephropathy.

Alpha cell: is a type of cell in the islets of Langerhans of the pancreas. They make and release the hormone glucagon when blood glucose falls too low. Glucagon then directs the liver to release glucose into the blood for energy, thereby preventing hypoglycemia in diabetic patients.

Alpha-glucosidase inhibitor: is a class of oral medicine for Type 2 diabetes. It blocks the enzymes that digest starches in food, resulting in a slower rise in blood glucose throughout the day. E.g., Acarbose (Precose) and Miglitol (Glycet).

Allopurinol: is a drug prescribed to bring down levels of uric acid. It also slows down the rate of kidney damage in patients with chronic renal disease. E.g., Riloric, Urid, Zyloric.

Amylin: is a peptide hormone formed by the beta cells in the pancreas. It regulates the timing of glucose release into the bloodstream after eating by slowing down the emptying process of the stomach. E.g., Pramlintide.

Amyotrophy: is a type of neuropathy that results in pain, weakness, and muscle wastage. It affects the thighs, hips, buttocks, and legs and causes weakness and wasting of pelvifemoral muscles.

Anaemia: is a condition in which the number of red blood cells is less than normal, resulting in less oxygen being carried to the body's cells. It results in low hemoglobin levels. The blood lacks sufficient amount of healthy red blood cells.

Angiopathy: is any disease of the blood vessels (veins, arteries, and capillaries). It is of two types—microangiopathy and macroangiopathy.

Antibodies: are proteins made by the body to protect itself from 'foreign' substances such as bacteria or viruses. Generally, antibodies help the body fight disease. However, people can get Type 1 diabetes when their bodies make antibodies that destroy the body's own insulin-making beta cells.

ARB: or Angiotensin Receptor Blocker is an oral medicine that lowers blood pressure. E.g., Candez, Lostat, Amchek-Z.

Arteriosclerosis: is the hardening, thickening, and loss of elasticity of the walls of the arteries. Arteriosclerosis is generally a heart problem but it can affect arteries in any other part of the body.

Artery: is a large blood vessel that carries blood with oxygen from the heart to all parts of the body.

Arrhythmia: is the abnormal beating of the heart which may be too slow (bradycardia), too fast (tachycardia), or irregular.

Aspart insulin: is a man-made form of human insulin. Its action is rapid. It starts to lower blood glucose within 10–20 minutes after injection. It has its strongest effect one to three hours after injection but keeps working for three to five hours after injection. E.g., NovoRapid, Novomix-30.

Aspartame: is a dietary sweetener with practically no calories and no nutritional value. Its safety is still being debated worldwide.

Atherosclerosis: is the clogging, narrowing, and hardening of the body's large arteries and medium-sized blood vessels. Atherosclerosis can lead to stroke, heart attack, eye problems, and kidney problems.

Autoimmune disease: is a disorder of the body's immune system in which the immune system mistakenly attacks and destroys body tissue that it believes to be foreign. E.g., Type 1 diabetes, Celiac disease or sprue, Hashimoto's thyroiditis, rheumatoid arthritis.

Autonomic neuropathy: is a type of neuropathy affecting the lungs, heart, stomach, intestines, bladder, or genitals. Diabetic Autonomic Neuropathy (DAN) can have the following manifestations: tachycardia or high heart beat, exercise intolerance, impaired functioning of the neurovascular system, constipation, erectile dysfunction, and brittle diabetes.

B

Background retinopathy (non-proliferative retinopathy): is a type of damage to the retina of the eye. It manifests as bleeding, fluid accumulation, and abnormal dilation of the blood vessels.

Bariatric surgery: from the Greek word 'baros' meaning 'weight', is synonymous with weight-loss surgery. The different types include Roux-en-y Gastric Bypass (RYGB), Biliopancreatic Diversion Surgery, Sleeve Gastrectomy, and Gastric Banding.

Basal rate: is the background insulin needed throughout the day to maintain the target glucose levels when a diabetic on an insulin pump is not eating food. It is a steady trickle of low levels of longer-acting insulin needed to prevent both hypoglycemia as well as hyperglycemia.

Beta cell: is a cell that makes exogenous insulin. Beta cells are located in the islets of Langerhans of the pancreas.

Biguanide: is a class of oral medicine used to treat Type 2 diabetes. Biguanides lower blood glucose levels by reducing the amount of glucose produced by the liver and also by making the body respond better to insulin. E.g., Metformin, Glucophage.

Blood glucose: is the main sugar found in the blood. Glucose is the body's main source of energy. Glucose comes from carbohydrate-rich foods like cereals. Blood glucose is also called blood sugar.

Blood glucose level: is the amount of glucose present in a given sample amount of blood. It is measured in milligrams per decilitre or mg/dl. The blood glucose level keeps changing throughout the day and night. It is dependent on the type and amount of food eaten. Normal values for blood glucose after eight hours of fasting range between 70 and 100 mg/dl.

Blood glucose monitor: is a small, portable machine used by diabetics to check their blood glucose levels. This helps in proper diabetic management. After pricking the skin with a lancet, a drop of blood is placed on a test strip in the machine. The monitor soon displays the blood glucose level as a number on the monitor's digital display.

Blood glucose monitoring: is the checking of a diabetic patient's blood glucose level on a regular basis in order to manage his diabetes in a better way. A blood glucose monitor helps with this.

Blood pressure: is the force of blood exerted on the inside walls of blood vessels. Blood pressure is expressed as a ratio, e.g., 120/80 or 110/76 or 185/92, etc. The upper number is the systolic (maximum) pressure, or the pressure exerted when the heart pushes blood out into the arteries. The lower number is the diastolic (minimum) pressure, or the pressure exerted when the heart rests.

Blood urea nitrogen (BUN): is a waste product in the blood that results from the digestion of protein. When protein is broken down, urea is made in the liver. The kidneys filter blood to remove urea through the urine. As kidney function decreases, the BUN levels increase.

Blood vessels: are tubes that form a part of the circulatory system in the body. Blood vessels carry blood to and from all the different parts of the body. The three main types of blood vessels are arteries, veins, and capillaries. Other blood vessels include arterioles and venules.

Body Mass Index (BMI): is a measure used to evaluate body weight relative to a person's height. It is also called the Quetelet Index. BMI is used to find out if a person is underweight, normal weight, overweight, or obese.

Bolus insulin: is an extra amount of insulin (generally

rapid-acting) taken before mealtimes, to cover an expected rise in blood glucose after the consumption of a full meal or heavy snack. Some patients may be advised to take it during or immediately after a meal to prevent hypoglycemia from setting in.

Brittle diabetes: is mainly associated with Type 1 diabetes but can also affect poorly controlled Type 2 diabetics. It is a term used when a person's blood glucose level swings very often from hypoglycemia to hyperglycemia and vice versa.

Bunion: is a bulge on the outside edge of the first joint of the big toe, caused by the swelling of a fluid sac under the skin. It causes the big toe to point towards the second toe. This spot can become red, sore, and infected. It is commoner in women.

C

C-peptide: or connecting peptide is a substance that the pancreas releases into the bloodstream in equal amounts to insulin. A test of C-peptide levels shows exactly how much insulin the body is making. Insulin and C-peptide are both linked when made by the pancreas.

Callus: is a small area of skin, usually on the feet and hands, that has become thick and hard from rubbing or pressure. Calluses on the feet are more common because of the pressure exerted and friction caused when walking.

Calorie: is a unit used to show the energy provided by food. Carbohydrates, proteins, fats, and alcohol provide calories in the diet. Carbohydrates and proteins each provide 4 calories per gram, fats provide 9 calories per gm, and pure alcohol provides 7 calories per gram.

Capillary: is the smallest blood vessel of the body which plays a role in micro-circulation. Capillaries transport blood from arteries to veins. Oxygen and glucose pass through capillary walls and enter the cells. Waste products such as carbon dioxide pass back from the cells into the blood through capillaries.

Capsaicin: is an antioxidant found in fiery hot peppers. Habaneros have the most capsaicin, jalapenos have some, but bell peppers have none. Capsaicin is an ingredient that can be found in ointment form for use on the skin to relieve pain from diabetic neuropathy.

Carbohydrate: is one of the three main nutrients in food, the others being protein and fat. Foods that provide carbohydrate include cereals like rice and wheat, starches, vegetables, fruits, dairy products, and sugars. Diabetics need to watch their carbohydrate intake, especially the intake of simple carbohydrates like sugar.

Carbohydrate counting: is a method of meal planning for people with diabetes. It is based on counting the total number of grams of simple carbohydrate as well as complex carbohydrate in food.

Cardiac ablation: is a hospital procedure used to destroy small areas of the heart muscle that cause problems with heart rhythm. These problems include chest pain, sweating, palpitations, skipping of heartbeats, dizziness, and light-headedness.

Cardiologist: is a doctor who treats people who have heart problems like coronary artery disease, heart failure, etc.

Cardiometabolic risk factors: are a set of conditions like obesity, hypertension, hyperglycemia, dyslipidemia, etc. that have a bearing on whether or not a person develops Type 2 diabetes or heart disease.

Cardiovascular disease: is a disease of the heart and blood vessels (arteries, veins, and capillaries) and is associated with atherosclerosis. It includes heart valve disease, arrhythmia, heart attack, and stroke.

Cataract: is a form of vision impairment caused by the clouding of the lens of the eye. The cloudiness is caused by the build-up of protein in the lens. If spectacles do not help in correcting the vision, then surgery may be required to remove the cloudy lens and replace it with an artificial one.

Cerebrovascular disease: is the damage to blood vessels in the brain. These vessels can burst and bleed or become clogged with fatty deposits. When blood flow is interrupted, the brain cells die or are damaged, resulting in a stroke.

Charcot's foot: is a condition in which the bones, joints, and soft tissue in the foot and ankle are deformed and destroyed. It results from damage to the nerves and cause 'rocker bottom' foot.

Chlorpropamide: is a sulfonylurea oral medication used to treat Type 2 diabetes. It lowers blood glucose levels by helping the pancreas make more insulin and by helping the body better use the insulin it makes. E.g., Copamide, Diabenese.

Cholesterol: is a type of fat produced by the liver and found in the blood that helps to make Vitamin D and hormones, and to build cell walls. Food sources include egg yolks, milk and milk products, meat, fish, poultry, etc. which have high levels of LDL cholesterol and low levels of HDL cholesterol and are associated with heart disease.

Chronic: describes something that lasts long, for more than three months, e.g., chronic renal disease, chronic respiratory disease, cancer.

Circulation: is the flow of blood through the body's blood vessels and heart.

Coma: is a sleep-like state in which a person is not conscious. Diabetic coma may be caused by hyperglycemia or hypoglycemia. It can be fatal.

Combination therapy: is a form of therapy for Type 2 diabetic patients which involves the use of different medicines together to manage their blood glucose levels better. E.g., a combination of different types of oral hypoglycemic agents or a combination of oral hypoglycemic agent and insulin.

Complications: are the harmful effects of diabetes such as damage to the eyes, heart, kidneys, blood vessels, nervous system, teeth, gums, feet, and skin. Keeping a tight control on blood glucose, blood pressure, and LDL cholesterol levels can help prevent or delay the onset of these problems.

Congenital defects: are problems or conditions that a child is born with, e.g., congenital heart disease.

Congestive heart failure: is the loss of the heart's pumping power, which causes fluids to collect in the body, especially in the feet and lungs. It causes shortness of breath, weakness, and swelling.

Coronary heart disease: is a type of heart disease caused by narrowing of the arteries that supply blood to the heart. If the blood supply is cut off, the result is a heart attack. This can be fatal if not attended to on time.

Creatinine: is a waste product from protein in the diet and from the muscles of the body. Creatinine is removed from the body by the kidneys. A high-protein diet increases the load on the kidneys. If the kidneys are malfunctioning, kidney disease progresses and the level of creatinine in the blood increases. This can lead to renal failure, necessitating dialysis or a kidney transplant.

D

D-phenylalanine derivative: is a class of oral medicine used in the treatment of Type 2 diabetes. It lowers blood glucose levels by helping the pancreas make more insulin immediately after meals. E.g., Glinate, Natiz.

Dawn phenomenon: is the early-morning (2–8 am) rise in the blood glucose level. The liver can release glucose at the time when growth hormones, cortisol, etc. are being released.

Dehydration: is the loss of too much body fluid through frequent urinating, sweating, diarrhoea, or vomiting. Dehydration can kill faster than starvation.

Dermopathy: is a disease of the skin. It results in reddish, oval scaly patches on the shins. Diabetic dermopathy can manifest in patients who have had diabetes for more than 20 years.

Desensitization: is a way to reduce or stop an allergic reaction to something. E.g., if a diabetic has an allergic reaction to a type of insulin, then his diabetologist will prescribe a very small amount of that insulin at first to increase his tolerance. Over a period of time, larger doses are given until the patient is taking the full dose. This is one way to help the body get used to the full dose and to prevent the allergic reaction.

Dextrose or glucose: is the simple sugar found in blood that serves as the body's main source of energy. It is derived from carbohydrates in food. It is the only form of energy that will energize the brain.

Diabetes educator: is a certified healthcare professional who teaches diabetic patients more about their disease and how to best manage their condition.

Diabetes insipidus: is a condition characterized by frequent and heavy urination, excessive thirst, and an overall feeling of weakness. This condition may be caused by a defect in the pituitary gland or in the kidney. Unlike in diabetes mellitus, in diabetes insipidus, blood glucose levels are normal.

Diabetes mellitus: is a condition characterized by hyperglycemia resulting from the body's inability to use blood glucose for energy. In Type 1 diabetes, the pancreas no longer makes insulin and therefore blood glucose cannot enter the cells to be used for energy. In Type 2 diabetes, either the pancreas does not make enough insulin or the body is unable to use this insulin correctly.

Diabetic diarrhoea: is a condition characterized by loose stools and faecal incontinence. It may result from an overgrowth of bacteria in the small intestine and also from intestinal diabetic neuropathy. The intestinal nerve damage can also result in constipation.

Diabetic ketoacidosis (DKA): is an emergency condition in which extremely high blood glucose levels, along with a severe lack of insulin, result in the breakdown of body fat for energy and an accumulation of ketones in the blood and urine. Signs of DKA are nausea and vomiting, stomach pain, fruity or acetone-like breath, and rapid breathing. If not treated on time, DKA can lead to coma and death.

Diabetic mastopathy: is a rare fibrous breast condition occurring in women, and sometimes men, with long-standing diabetes. The lumps are not malignant and can be surgically removed, although they often recur.

Diabetic myelopathy: is the damage to the spinal cord caused by lesions. It is found in some people with diabetes.

Diabetic retinopathy: is a form of eye disease in diabetics with poor blood glucose control. It results in damage to the small blood vessels in the retina. If not treated on time, it can lead to blindness.

Diabetogenic: is a term used to describe something that causes diabetes, e.g., thiazide diuretics and beta blockers that reduce blood pressure, corticosteroids prescribed to reduce inflammation.

Diabetologist: is a doctor who specializes in treating people with diabetes.

Diagnosis: is the determination of a disease from its signs and symptoms.

Dialysis: is the process of cleaning waste from the blood artificially. This job is normally done by the kidneys. If the kidneys fail, the blood must be cleaned artificially with special equipment. The two major forms of dialysis are hemodialysis and peritoneal dialysis.

Dietitian: is a healthcare professional who advises people about meal planning, food exchanges, calorie counting, weight control, and diabetes management.

Dilated eye exam: is a test done by an eyecare specialist in which the pupil of the eye is temporarily enlarged with eyedrops to allow the specialist to see the inside of the eye more easily.

Dupuytren's contracture: is a condition associated with diabetes. It affects the tissue below the skin of the palms of the hands. The fingers and the palm of the hand gradually thicken and shorten, leading the fingers to curve inward.

E

Electromyography (EMG): is a test used to detect nerve function. It measures the electrical activity generated by muscles.

Endocrine gland: is a group of specialized cells that release hormones into the blood. For example, the islets in the pancreas, which secrete insulin, are endocrine glands. Other examples include adrenal glands, thyroid gland, ovaries, testes, pituitary glands, etc.

Endocrinologist: is a doctor who treats people who have endocrine gland problems such as diabetes, thyroid disease, etc.

Enzyme: is a complex protein made by the body that helps to bring about a chemical reaction in the body. Enzymes are made in the blood, intestinal fluids, mouth, and stomach. They have a specificity of action: amylases help in carbohydrate digestion, lipases aid in fat digestion, and proteases help in protein digestion. E.g., the enzyme made in the mouth is the salivary enzyme called salivary amylase or ptyalin which helps in carbohydrate digestion.

Euglycemia: is a normal level of glucose in the blood. It is generally between 70 and 100 mg/dl for a fasting blood sample.

Exchange lists: are one of several approaches for diabetes meal planning. Foods are categorized into three groups based on their nutritional content. Lists provide the serving sizes for carbohydrates, meat and meat alternatives, and fats. These lists allow for substitution for different groups to keep the nutritional content fixed.

Endogenous insulin: is the insulin produced within the human body. It is secreted by the beta cells of the islets of Langerhans of the pancreas.

Exogenous insulin: is the insulin produced by sources other than the human body. It has to be injected into the subcutaneous layer of the skin of the diabetic patient, e.g. bovine insulin, porcine insulin, and recombinant human insulin.

F

Fasting blood glucose test: is a check of a person's blood glucose level after the person has not eaten for 8–12 hours. It is generally done after a period of overnight fasting. This test is used to diagnose pre-diabetes and diabetes. It is also used to monitor people with diabetes.

Fat: is one of the three main nutrients in food which energize the body. Each gram of fat provides 9 calories of energy. Foods that provide fat are ghee, butter, margarine, salad dressing, oil, nuts, meat, poultry, fish, and dairy products like milk and cream. Excess calories are stored as body fat in the adipose tissue. They provide the body with a reserve supply of energy.

Fluorescein angiography: is a test used to examine the blood vessels in the eye. It is done by injecting a dye into an arm vein and then taking photos as the dye goes through the eye's blood vessels.

Fructosamine test: is a measure of the number of blood glucose molecules linked to protein molecules in the blood. The test provides information about the average blood glucose level for the past three weeks. It is a good indicator of blood glucose management.

Fructose: is a sugar that occurs naturally in fruits and honey. Fructose has 4 calories per gram.

G

Gangrene: is the term used to indicate the death of body tissue. It is most often caused by a lack of blood flow to a limb and by infection. It can lead to amputation.

Gastroparesis: is a form of neuropathy that affects the stomach muscles. Digestion of food may be incomplete or delayed because of this, resulting in gas formation, abdominal bloating, nausea, or vomiting. A diabetic with gastroparesis experiences difficulty in controlling his blood glucose levels.

Gestational diabetes mellitus (GDM): is a type of diabetes mellitus that develops only during pregnancy and usually disappears upon delivery, but increases the risk of the mother developing diabetes later on in life. GDM must be managed with diet control, moderate exercise, oral hypoglycemics, or insulin.

Gingivitis: is a condition of the gums characterized by inflammation and bleeding. Since diabetes affects the body's ability to use blood sugar, patients with this disease are at higher risk of developing infections, including periodontal disease and cavities. If not treated, it can lead to periodontitis or gum disease.

Gland: is a group of cells that secrete substances. Endocrine glands secrete hormones like insulin. Exocrine glands secrete salt, enzymes, and water.

Glargine insulin: is a very long-acting insulin. Glargine insulin starts to lower blood glucose levels within one hour after injection and keeps working evenly for 24 hours after injection. It is injected subcutaneously once a day, preferably at the same time each day. E.g., Lantus and Humalog.

Glaucoma: is an increase in fluid pressure inside the eye that may lead to loss of vision.

Glimepiride: is a sulfonylurea oral medicine used to treat Type 2 diabetes. It lowers blood glucose by helping the pancreas make more insulin and by helping the body better use the insulin it makes. E.g. Amaryl.

Glipizide: is a sulfonylurea oral medicine used to treat Type 2 diabetes. It lowers blood glucose by helping the pancreas make more insulin and by helping the body better use the insulin it makes. E.g., Diaglip, Glucotrol, Glynase.

Glomerular filtration rate (GFR): is a measure of the kidney's ability to filter and remove waste products. It is checked to find out if a person is suffering from kidney disease.

Glomerulus: is a tiny set of looping blood vessels in the kidney where the blood is filtered and waste products are removed.

Glucagon: is a hormone produced by the alpha cells in the pancreas. It raises blood glucose levels. An injectable form of glucagon may be used to treat cases of severe hypoglycemia.

Glucose: is one of the simplest forms of sugar. When food is consumed, the carbohydrates in food are converted into glucose. This glucose is then utilized for energy or stored in the cells for future use.

Glucose tablets: are chewable tablets made of pure glucose used for treating hypoglycemia.

Glucovance: is an oral medicine used to treat Type 2 diabetes. It is a combination of glyburide and metformin.

Glyburide: is a sulfonylurea oral medicine used to treat Type 2 diabetes. It lowers blood glucose by helping the pancreas make more insulin and by helping the body better use the insulin it makes. E.g., DiaBeta, Glynase. It is also an ingredient in Glucovance.

Glycemic Index (GI): is a ranking of carbohydrate-rich foods, based on the food's effect on blood glucose compared with a standard reference food (glucose). GI measures the impact of different foods on blood glucose levels.

Glycogen: is the storage form of glucose synthesized and stored in the liver and muscles. Diabetes leads to abnormal glycogen metabolism.

Glycosuria: is the presence of glucose in urine. It results from high blood glucose levels. Urine generally does not contain glucose.

Gram: is a unit of weight in the metric system. An ounce equals 28 gm. In many diabetic diets, the recommendations for amounts of food may be given in grams.

H

HbA1C: is a test that measures a person's average blood glucose level over the past two to three months. Haemoglobin is the part of a red blood cell that carries oxygen to the cells and sometimes joins with the glucose in the blood. Red blood cells typically live for three months. The test, which is also called A1C or glycosylated haemoglobin or glycohaemoglobin test, shows the amount of glucose that adheres to the red blood cell. This is proportional to the amount of glucose in the blood.

HDL cholesterol (high-density lipoprotein cholesterol): is a fat found in the blood that takes extra cholesterol from the blood to the liver for removal. It is sometimes called 'good' cholesterol because it reduces the risk of heart disease.

Heredity: is the passing of a trait from one generation to another of from parent to child. This results in children looking like their parents or in siblings resembling one another.

Honeymoon phase: Some people with Type 1 diabetes experience a brief remission called the 'honeymoon period'. During this time, their pancreas may still secrete some insulin. Over time, this secretion stops and, as this happens, the person will require more insulin from injections. The honeymoon period can last weeks, months, or even up to a year or more.

Hormone: is a chemical produced in one part of the body and released into the blood to trigger or regulate particular functions of the body. For example, insulin is a hormone made in the pancreas which tells other cells when to use glucose for energy. Other examples include estrogen, progesterone, testosterone, cortisol, leptin, etc.

Human leukocyte antigens (HLA): are proteins located on the surface of the cell that help the immune system identify the cell either as one belonging to the body or as one from outside the body. Some patterns of these proteins may mean increased risk of developing Type 1 diabetes.

Hyperglycemia: is a condition resulting in excessive blood glucose. Fasting hyperglycemia is blood glucose above a desirable level after a person has fasted for at least eight hours. Postprandial hyperglycemia is blood glucose above a desirable level two hours after a person has eaten.

Hyperinsulinemia: is a condition in which the level of insulin in the blood is higher than normal. It is generally caused by overproduction of insulin in the body. It is related to insulin resistance.

Hyperlipidemia: is a condition in which the body has higher than normal fat and cholesterol levels in the blood.

Hyperosmolar hyperglycemic nonketotic syndrome (HHNS): is an emergency condition in which the diabetic patient's blood glucose level is very high and ketones are not present in the blood or urine. If HHNS is not treated, it can lead to coma or death.

Hypertension: is a condition that occurs when blood flows through the blood vessels with a force greater than normal. It is also called high blood pressure. Hypertension can strain the heart, damage the blood vessels, and increase the risk of heart attack, stroke, kidney problems, and death.

Hypoglycemia: is a condition that occurs when the patient's blood glucose level is lower than normal, usually less than 70 mg/dl. Signs include hunger, nervousness, shakiness, perspiration, dizziness or light-headedness, sleepiness, and confusion. If left untreated, hypoglycemia may lead to unconsciousness. Hypoglycemia is treated by consuming a carbohydrate-rich food such as a glucose tablet or juice. It may also be treated with an injection of glucagon if the person is unconscious or unable to swallow. This can be the result of an insulin reaction.

Hypoglycemia unawareness: is a state in which a person does not feel or recognize the symptoms of hypoglycemia. People who have frequent episodes of hypoglycemia may no longer experience the warning signs of it.

Hypotension: is the condition of low blood pressure or a sudden drop in blood pressure. Hypotension may occur when a person rises quickly from a sitting or reclining position, causing dizziness or fainting.

I

IDDM: is the former term for Type 1 diabetes.

Immune system: is the body's system for protecting itself from viruses and bacteria or any 'foreign' substances.

Imunosuppressant: is a drug that suppresses the natural immune responses. Immunosuppressants are given to transplant patients to prevent organ rejection or to patients with autoimmune diseases.

Impaired fasting glucose (IFG): is a condition in which a blood glucose test, taken after an 8–12 hour fast, shows a level of glucose higher than normal but not high enough for a diagnosis of diabetes. IFG, also called pre-diabetes, is a level of 100 mg/dL to 125 mg/dl. Most people with pre-diabetes are at increased risk for developing Type 2 diabetes. They should be careful about their diet and increase their exercise pattern.

Impaired glucose tolerance (IGT): is a condition in which blood glucose levels are higher than normal but are not high enough for a diagnosis of diabetes. IGT, also called pre-diabetes, is a level of 140 mg/dL to 199 mg/dl two hours after the start of an oral glucose tolerance test. Most people with pre-diabetes are at increased risk for developing Type 2 diabetes. IGT was previously known as borderline diabetes.

Implantable insulin pump: is a small pump placed inside the body to deliver insulin in response to remote-control commands from the user.

Impotence: is the inability to get or maintain an erection for sexual activity. It is also called erectile dysfunction (ED). Diabetic males are more prone to ED than non-diabetic males.

Incidence: is a measure of how often a disease occurs; the number of new cases of a disease among a certain group of people for a certain period of time. E.g., the incidence of diabetes is higher in the Indian subcontinent.

Incontinence: is loss of bladder or bowel control resulting in the accidental discharge of urine or faeces. It can be of different types like stress incontinence, urge incontinence, functional incontinence, etc.

Inhaled insulin: is an experimental treatment for taking insulin using a portable device that allows a person to breathe in insulin.

Injection: is the process of inserting liquid medication or nutrients into the body with a syringe. A person with diabetes may use short needles or pinch the skin and inject at an angle to avoid an intramuscular injection of insulin.

Injection site rotation: is the changing of the places on the body where insulin is injected. Rotation prevents the formation of lipodystrophies. A lipodystrophy is a lump formed in the skin when insulin is injected in the same spot.

Injection sites: are the places on the body where insulin is usually injected. E.g., stomach, outer side of the upper thighs, back of the upper arms, buttocks, hips, etc.

Insulin: is a hormone made by the beta cells of the islets of Langerhans of the pancreas that helps the body use glucose for energy. When the body cannot make enough insulin, it is taken by injection or through use of an insulin pump.

Insulin adjustment: is a change in the amount of insulin a person with diabetes takes based on factors such as meal intake, activity, and blood glucose levels.

Insulin analogues: is a tailored form of insulin in which certain amino acids in the insulin molecule have been modified. The analogue acts in the same way as the original insulin, but with some beneficial differences for people with diabetes.

Insulin pen: is a device for injecting insulin that looks like a fountain pen and holds replaceable cartridges of insulin. It is also available in disposable form.

Insulin pump: is an insulin-delivering device about the size of a deck of cards that can be worn on a belt or kept in a pocket. An insulin pump connects to a narrow, flexible plastic tubing that ends with a needle inserted just under the skin. Users set the pump to give a steady trickle or basal amount of insulin continuously throughout the day. Pumps release bolus doses of insulin (several units at a time) at meals and at times when blood glucose is too high, based on programming done by the user.

Insulin reaction: is a condition which occurs when the level of glucose in the blood is too low (at or below 70 mg/dl). It is also known as hypoglycemia.

Insulin receptors: are areas on the outer part of a cell that allow the cell to bind with insulin in the blood. When the cell and insulin bind, the cell can take glucose from the blood and use it for energy.

Insulin resistance: is the body's inability to respond to and use the insulin it produces. Insulin resistance may be linked to obesity, hypertension, and high levels of fat in the blood.

Insulin-dependent diabetes mellitus (IDDM): is the former term for Type 1 diabetes.

Insulinoma: is a tumour of the beta cells in the pancreas. An insulinoma may cause the body to make extra insulin, leading to hypoglycemia.

Intensive therapy: is a treatment for diabetes in which

blood glucose is kept as close to normal as possible through frequent injections or use of an insulin pump, meal planning, adjustment of medicines, and exercise based on blood glucose test results and frequent contact with a person's healthcare team.

Intermediate-acting insulin: is a type of insulin that starts to lower blood glucose within one to two hours after injection and has its strongest effect six to twelve hours after injection, depending on the type used. E.g., lente insulin and NPH (neutral protamine Hagedorn) insulin.

Intermittent claudication: is a type of pain that comes and goes in the muscles of the leg. This pain results from a lack of blood supply to the legs and usually happens when walking or exercising.

Intramuscular injection: is the insertion of liquid medication into a muscle with a syringe. E.g., glucagon may be given by subcutaneous or intramuscular injection for hypoglycemia.

Inulin: is a starchy substance found in chicory roots, wheat, onions, bananas, leeks, artichokes, and asparagus. It is used for high blood fats (cholesterol and triglycerides). It is also used for weight loss and constipation. Since it is not digested or absorbed in the stomach, it goes to the bowels where it supports the growth of a special kind of bacteria that is associated with improving bowel function and general health. Inulin decreases the body's ability to make certain kinds of fats.

Islet cell autoantibodies (ICA): are proteins found in the blood of people newly diagnosed with Type 1 diabetes. They are also found in people who may be developing Type 1 diabetes. The presence of ICA indicates that the body's immune system has been damaging the beta cells in the pancreas.

Islet transplantation: is a process involving the moving of the islets from a donor pancreas into a person whose pancreas has stopped producing insulin. Beta cells in the islets make the insulin that the body needs for using blood glucose.

Islets: are groups of cells located in the pancreas that make hormones that help the body break down and use food. For example, alpha cells make glucagon and beta cells make insulin. They are also called islets of Langerhans.

J

Jet injector: is a device that uses high pressure instead of a needle to propel insulin through the skin and into the body.

Juvenile diabetes: is the former term for insulin-dependent diabetes mellitus (IDDM) or Type 1 diabetes.

K

Ketone: is a chemical produced when there is a shortage of insulin in the blood and the body breaks down body fat for energy. High levels of ketones can lead to diabetic ketoacidosis and coma. It can be fatal.

Ketonuria: is a condition occurring when ketones are present in the urine, a warning sign of diabetic ketoacidosis.

Ketosis: is a ketone build-up in the body that may lead to diabetic ketoacidosis. The general signs of ketosis are nausea, vomiting, and stomach pain.

Kidney failure: is a chronic condition in which the body retains fluid and harmful wastes build-up because the kidneys no longer work properly. A person with kidney failure needs dialysis or a kidney transplant. It is also called end-stage renal disease or ESRD.

Kidneys: are the two bean-shaped organs that filter wastes from the blood and form urine. The kidneys are located near the middle of the back. They send urine to the bladder.

Kussmaul breathing: is the rapid, deep, and laboured breathing of people who have diabetic ketoacidosis.

L

Lancet: is a spring-loaded device used to prick the skin with a small needle to obtain a drop of blood for blood glucose monitoring.

Laser surgery treatment: is a type of therapy that uses a strong beam of light to treat a damaged area. The beam of light is called a laser. A laser is sometimes used to seal blood vessels in the eye of a person with diabetes.

Latent autoimmune diabetes in adults (LADA): is a condition in which Type 1 diabetes develops in adults.

LDL cholesterol (low-density lipoprotein cholesterol): is a fat found in the blood that takes cholesterol around the body to where it is needed for cell repair and also deposits it on the inside of artery walls. It is sometimes called 'bad' cholesterol because it increases the risk of heart disease.

Lente insulin: is an intermediate-acting insulin. On an average, lente insulin starts to lower blood glucose levels within one to two hours after injection. It has its strongest effect 8–12 hours after injection but keeps working for 18–24 hours after injection.

Limited joint mobility: is a condition in which the joints swell up and the skin of the hand becomes thick, tight, and waxy, making the joints less able to move. It may affect the fingers and arms as well as other joints in the body.

Lipid: is a term for fat in the body. Lipids can be broken down by the body and used for energy. Each gram of lipid provides the body with 9 calories of energy.

Lipid profile: is a blood test that measures total cholesterol, triglycerides, HDL cholesterol, LDL cholesterol, and VLDL (very-low-density lipoprotein) cholesterol. A lipid profile is one of the measures of a person's risk of cardiovascular disease.

Lipoatrophy: is the loss of fat under the skin resulting in small dents. Lipoatrophy may be caused by repeated injections of insulin in the same spot.

Lipodystrophy: is a defect in the breaking down or building up of fat below the surface of the skin, resulting in lumps or small dents in the skin surface. Lipodystrophy may be caused by repeated injections of insulin in the same spot.

Lipohypertrophy: is the build-up of fat below the surface of the skin, causing lumps. Lipohypertrophy may be caused by repeated injections of insulin in the same spot.

Lispro insulin: is a rapid-acting insulin. On average, lispro insulin starts to lower blood glucose within five minutes after injection. It has its strongest effect 30 minutes to one hour after injection but keeps working for three hours after injection. E.g., Humalog, NovoRapid.

Liver: is an organ in the body that changes food into energy, removes alcohol and poisons from the blood, and makes bile, a substance that breaks down fats and helps rid the body of wastes.

Long-acting insulin: is a type of insulin that starts to lower blood glucose within four to six hours after injection and has its strongest effect ten to eighteen hours after injection. E.g., Ultralente insulin.

M

Macrosomia: is a term used to indicate abnormally large babies that may be born to women with diabetes.

Macrovascular disease: is a disease of the large blood vessels, such as those found in the heart. Lipids and blood clots build up in the large blood vessels and can cause atherosclerosis, coronary heart disease, stroke, and peripheral vascular disease.

Macula: is the part of the retina in the eye used for reading and seeing fine detail.

Macular Oedema: is the swelling of the macula.

Maturity-onset diabetes of the young (MODY): is a kind of Type 2 diabetes that accounts for 1–5 per cent of people with diabetes.

Meglitinide: is a class of oral medicine for Type 2 diabetes that lowers blood glucose by helping the pancreas make more insulin right after meals. E.g., Repaglinide.

Metabolic syndrome: is the tendency of several conditions to occur together, including obesity, insulin resistance, diabetes or pre-diabetes, hypertension, and high lipids.

Metabolism: is the term for the way cells chemically change food so that it can be used to store or use energy and make the proteins, fats, and sugars needed by the body.

Metformin: is a biguanide oral medicine used to treat Type 2 diabetes. It lowers blood glucose by reducing the amount of glucose produced by the liver and helping the body respond better to the insulin made in the pancreas. E.g., Glucophage, Glucophage XR.\

Mg/dl: or milligrams per decilitre is a unit of measurement that shows the concentration of a substance in a specific amount of fluid. Generally, blood glucose test results are reported as mg/dl.

Microalbumin: is the detection of small amounts of the protein called albumin in the urine. It is detectable with a special laboratory test.

Microalbuminuria: is the presence of small amounts of albumin, a protein, in the urine. Microalbuminuria is an early sign of kidney damage, or nephropathy, a common and serious complication of diabetes. The ADA (American Diabetes Association) recommends that people diagnosed with Type 2 diabetes be tested for microalbuminuria at the time they are diagnosed and every year thereafter; people with Type 1 diabetes should be tested five years after diagnosis and every year thereafter. Microalbuminuria is usually managed by improving blood glucose control, reducing blood pressure, and modifying the diet.

Microaneurysm: is a small swelling that forms on the side of tiny blood vessels. These swellings may break and allow blood to leak into nearby tissue. People with diabetes may get microaneurysms in the retina of the eye.

Microvascular disease: is a disease of the smallest blood vessels, such as those found in the eyes, nerves, and kidneys. The walls of the vessels become abnormally thick but weak. Then they bleed, leak protein, and slow the flow of blood to the cells.

Miglitol: is an alpha-glucosidase inhibitor oral medicine used to treat Type 2 diabetes. It blocks the enzymes that digest starches in food. The result is a slower and lower rise in blood glucose throughout the day, especially right after meals. E.g., Glyset.

Mixed dose: is a combination of two types of insulin in one injection. Usually a rapid- or short-acting insulin is combined with a longer acting insulin (such as NPH insulin) to provide both short-term and long-term control of blood glucose levels.

Mmol/l: or millimoles per litre is a unit of measure that shows the concentration of a substance in a specific amount of fluid.

Monofilament: is a short piece of nylon, like a hairbrush bristle, mounted on a wand. To check sensitivity of the nerves in the foot, the doctor touches the filament to the bottom of the foot.

Mononeuropathy: is a type of neuropathy affecting a single nerve.

Myocardial infarction: is an interruption in the blood supply to the heart because of narrowed or blocked blood vessels. It is also called a heart attack.

N

Nateglinide: is a D-phenylalanine derivative oral medicine used to treat Type 2 diabetes. It lowers blood glucose levels by helping the pancreas make more insulin right after meals. E.g., Starlix.

Necrobiosis lipoidica diabeticorum: is a skin condition usually on the lower part of the legs. Lesions can be small or extend over a large area. They are usually raised, yellow, and waxy in appearance and often have a purple border.

Neovascularization: is the growth of new, small blood vessels. In the retina, this may lead to loss of vision or blindness.

Nephrologist: is a doctor who treats people who have kidney problems.

Nephropathy: is a disease of the kidneys. Hyperglycemia and hypertension can damage the kidneys' glomeruli. When the kidneys are damaged, protein leaks out of the kidneys into the urine. Damaged kidneys can no longer remove waste and extra fluids from the bloodstream.

Nerve conduction studies: is a series of tests used to measure for nerve damage. It is one way to diagnose neuropathy.

Neurologist: is a doctor who specializes in problems of the nervous system, such as neuropathy.

Neuropathy: is a disease of the nervous system. The three major forms in people with diabetes are peripheral neuropathy, autonomic neuropathy, and mononeuropathy. The most common form is peripheral neuropathy, which affects mainly the legs and feet.

NIDDM: or noninsulin-dependent diabetes mellitus is the former term for Type 2 diabetes.

Non-invasive blood glucose monitoring: is a method of measuring blood glucose without pricking the finger to obtain a blood sample.

NPH insulin: is an intermediate-acting insulin. NPH stands for neutral protamine Hagedorn. On average, NPH insulin starts to lower blood glucose within one to two hours after injection. It has its strongest effect six to ten hours after injection but keeps working about ten hours after injection. It is also called N insulin.

Nutritionist: is a person with training in nutrition who advises on matters of food.

O

Obesity: is a condition in which a greater than normal amount of fat is in the body. It is more severe than being overweight. An obese individual is one having a body mass index (BMI) of 30 or more.

Obstetrician: is a doctor who treats pregnant women and delivers babies.

Oedema: is the swelling caused by excess fluid in the body. It results when small blood vessels release fluid into nearby tissues. This extra fluid accumulates, causing the tissue to swell.

Ophthalmologist: is a medical doctor who diagnoses and treats all eye diseases and eye disorders. Opthalmologists can also prescribe glasses and contact lenses.

Optician: is a healthcare professional who dispenses glasses and lenses. An optician also makes and fits contact lenses.

Optometrist: is a primary eye care provider who prescribes glasses and contact lenses. Optometrists can diagnose and treat certain eye conditions and diseases.

OGTT: or oral glucose tolerance test is a test to diagnose pre-diabetes and diabetes. The oral glucose tolerance test is given by a health care professional after an overnight fast. A blood sample is taken after which the patient drinks a high-glucose beverage. Blood samples are taken at intervals for two to three hours. Test results are compared with a standard and show how the body uses glucose over time.

OHAs-oral hypoglycemic agents: is a term used to describe medicines taken by mouth by people with Type 2 diabetes to keep blood glucose levels as close to normal as possible. Classes of oral hypoglycemic agents are alpha-glucosidase inhibitors, biguanides, D-phenylalanine derivatives, meglitinides, sulfonylureas, and thiazolidinediones.

Overweight: is a term used to describe an individual with an above-normal body weight. An overweight individual has a body mass index of 25 to 29.9.

P

Pancreas: is an organ that makes insulin and enzymes for digestion. It is located behind the lower part of the stomach and is about the size of a hand.

Pancreas transplantation: is a surgical procedure to take a healthy whole or partial pancreas from a donor and place it into the body of a person with diabetes.

Pediatric endocrinologist: is a doctor who treats children who have endocrine gland problems such as diabetes and thyroid issues.

Pedorthist: is a healthcare professional who specializes in fitting shoes for people with disabilities or deformities. A pedorthist can custom-make shoes or orthotics (special inserts for shoes).

Periodontal disease: is a disease of the gums.

Periodontist: is a dentist who specializes in treating people who have gum diseases.

Peripheral neuropathy: is the nerve damage that affects the feet, legs, or hands. Peripheral neuropathy causes pain, numbness, or a burning or tingling feeling.

PVD: or peripheral vascular disease is a disease of the large blood vessels of the arms, legs, and feet. PVD may occur when major blood vessels in these areas are blocked and do not receive enough blood. The signs of PVD are aching pains and slow-healing foot sores.

Pharmacist: is a healthcare professional who prepares and distributes medicine to people. Pharmacists also give information on medicines.

Photocoagulation: is a treatment for diabetic retinopathy. A strong beam of laser light is used to seal off bleeding blood vessels in the eye and to burn away extra blood vessels that should not have grown there.

Pioglitazone: is a thiazolidinedione oral medicine used to treat Type 2 diabetes. It helps insulin take glucose from the blood into the cells for energy by making cells more sensitive to insulin.

Podiatrist: is a doctor who treats people who have foot problems. Podiatrists also help people keep their feet healthy by providing regular foot examinations and treatment. Diabetics should regularly visit a podiatrist for their foot examinations.

Podiatry: is the care and treatment of feet.

Polydipsia: is the term used to describe excessive thirst which may be a sign of diabetes.

Polyphagia: is the term used to describe excessive hunger which may be a sign of diabetes.

Polyuria: is the term used to describe excessive urination which may be a sign of diabetes.

PPBS: or postprandial blood sugar is the blood glucose level taken two hours after eating a complete meal.

Pre-diabetes: is a condition in which blood glucose levels are higher than normal but are not high enough for a diagnosis of diabetes. People with pre-diabetes are at an increased risk for developing Type 2 diabetes and for heart disease and stroke. Other names for pre-diabetes are impaired glucose tolerance (IGT) and impaired fasting glucose. People with pre-diabetes should maintain a strict diet and exercise regimen.

Premixed insulin: is a commercially produced combination of two different types of insulin. E.g., 50:50 insulin, 75:25 insulin, and 70:30 insulin.

Pre-prandial blood glucose: is the blood glucose level taken before eating a meal. It is also called fasting blood glucose.

Prevalence: is the term used to describe the number of people in a given group or population who are reported to have a disease.

Proinsulin: is the pro-hormone precursor to insulin made first in the beta cells of the islets of Langerhans of the pancreas and then broken into several pieces to become insulin.

Proliferative retinopathy: is a condition in which tiny, fragile new blood vessels grow along the retina and in the vitreous humour of the eye.

Prosthesis: is a man-made substitute for a missing body part such as an arm or a leg. E.g., Jaipur foot.

Protein: is one of the main nutrients in food along with carbohydrates and fats. Foods that provide protein include meat, fish, poultry, dairy products like milk, paneer, cheese, dahi, mava, and khoya, eggs, lentils, and dried beans like soy beans and bean curd (tofu). Proteins are needed in the body for maintaining the cellular structure, producing hormones such as insulin, repairing wornout tissues and other functions. Each gram of protein provides the body with 4 calories of energy.

Proteinuria: is the presence of excess protein in the urine which can sometimes be the cause of foamy bubbles in the urine. It is indicative of malfunctioning kidneys.

R

Rapid-acting insulin: is a type of insulin that starts to lower blood glucose within five to ten minutes after injection and has its strongest effect thirty minutes to three hours after injection, depending on the type used.

Rebound hyperglycemia: is a swing to a high level of glucose in the blood after a low level.

Regular insulin: is a short-acting insulin. On average, regular insulin starts to lower blood glucose within thirty minutes after injection. It has its strongest effect two to five hours after injection but keeps working five to eight hours after injection.

Renal: is a term having to do with the kidneys. A renal disease is a disease of the kidneys. Renal failure means that the kidneys have stopped working.

Renal threshold of glucose: is the level of the blood glucose concentration at which the kidneys start to excrete glucose into the urine.

Repaglinide: is a meglitinide oral medicine used to treat Type 2 diabetes. It lowers blood glucose by helping the pancreas make more insulin right after meals. E.g., Prandin.

Retina: is the light-sensitive layer of tissue that lines the back of the eye.

Retinopathy: is the eye disease that is caused by damage to the small blood vessels in the retina. Diabetic retinopathy may result in loss of vision.

Risk factor: is a term used to describe anything that raises the chances of a person developing a disease.

Rosiglitazone: is a thiazolidinedione oral medicine used to treat Type 2 diabetes. It helps insulin take glucose from the blood into the cells for energy by making the cells more sensitive to insulin. E.g., Avandia.

S

Saccharin: is a sweetener with no calories and no nutritional value. Its use has been discontinued after it was found to be carcinogenic.

Secondary diabetes: is a type of diabetes caused by another disease or certain drugs or chemicals.

Self-management: in diabetes, is the ongoing process of managing diabetes. It includes meal planning, planned physical activity, blood glucose monitoring, taking diabetes medicines, handling episodes of illness and of low and high blood glucose, managing diabetes when travelling, and more. The person with diabetes designs his or her own self-management treatment plan in consultation with a variety of healthcare professionals such as doctors, nurses, dietitians, pharmacists, and others.

Sharps container: is a container for the disposal of used needles and syringes. It is often made of hard plastic so that needles cannot poke through.

Short-acting insulin: is a type of insulin that starts to lower blood glucose within thirty minutes after injection and has its strongest effect two to five hours after injection.

Side effects: are the unintended action(s) of a drug.

Sliding scale: is a set of instructions for adjusting insulin on the basis of blood glucose test results, meals, or activity levels.

Somogyi effect (rebound hyperglycemia): is a reaction which occurs when the blood glucose level swings high following hypoglycemia. The Somogyi effect may follow an untreated hypoglycemic episode during the night and is caused by the release of stress hormones like cortisol.

Sorbitol: is a sugar alcohol (sweetener) with 2.6 calories per gram. It is also a substance produced by the body in people with diabetes that can cause damage to the eyes and nerves.

Split mixed dose: is the division of a prescribed daily dose of insulin into two or more injections given over the course of the day.

Starch: is another name for carbohydrate, one of the three main nutrients in food. It is a storage form of carbohydrate in plant tissue.

Stroke: is a condition caused by damage to blood vessels in the brain. Strokes may cause loss of ability to speak or to move parts of the body.

Subcutaneous injection: is the process of putting a fluid into the tissue under the skin with a needle and syringe.

Sucralose: is a sweetener made from sugar but with no calories and no nutritional value.

Sucrose: is a two-part sugar made of glucose and fructose. Sucrose is known as table sugar or white sugar. It is found naturally in sugar cane and beet.

Sugar: is a class of carbohydrates with a sweet taste, including glucose, fructose, and sucrose. 'Sugar' is also a term used to refer to blood glucose.

Sugar alcohols: are sweeteners that produce a smaller rise in blood glucose than other carbohydrates. Their calorie content is about 2 calories per gram. Sugar alcohols include erythritol, hydrogenated starch hydrolysates, isomalt, lactitol, maltitol, mannitol, sorbitol, and xylitol. They are also known as polyols.

Sugar diabetes: is a former term for diabetes mellitus.

Sulfonylurea: is a class of oral medicine for Type 2 diabetes that lowers blood glucose by helping the pancreas make more insulin and by helping the body better use the insulin it makes. E.g., acetohexamide, chlorpropamide, glimepiride, glipizide, glyburide, tolazamide, tolbutamide.

Syringe: is a device used to inject medications or other liquids into body tissues. The syringe for insulin has a hollow plastic tube with a plunger inside and a needle on the end.

T

Tachycardia: is a condition in which the resting heart rate exceeds 100 beats per minute. This can disrupt the normal functioning of the heart. It can also increase the risk of cardiac arrest and stroke. Tachycardia can be fatal.

Team management: is a diabetes treatment approach in which medical care is provided by a team of healthcare professionals including a doctor, dietitian, nurse, diabetes educator, and others. The team acts as advisers to the person with diabetes.

Thiazolidinedione: is a class of oral medicine for Type 2 diabetes that helps insulin take glucose from the blood into the cells for energy by making cells more sensitive to insulin. E.g., pioglitazone, rosiglitazone.

Tolazamide: is a sulfonylurea oral medicine used to treat Type 2 diabetes. It lowers blood glucose by helping the pancreas make more insulin and by helping the body better use the insulin it makes. E.g., Tolinase.

Tolbutamide: is a sulfonylurea oral medicine used to treat Type 2 diabetes. It lowers blood glucose by helping the pancreas make more insulin and by helping the body better use the insulin it makes. E.g., Orinase.

Triglyceride: is the storage form of fat in the body. High triglyceride levels may occur when diabetes is out of control.

Type 1 diabetes: is a condition characterized by high blood glucose levels caused by a total lack of insulin. It occurs when the body's immune system attacks the insulin-producing beta cells in the pancreas and destroys them. The pancreas then produces little or no insulin. Type 1 diabetes develops most often in young people but can appear in adults.

Type 2 diabetes: is a condition characterized by high blood glucose levels caused by either a lack of insulin or the body's inability to use insulin efficiently. Type 2 diabetes develops most often in middle-aged and older adults but can appear in young people.

U

Ulcer: is a deep open sore or break in the skin. Diabetics' foot sores and ulcers can take several months to heal.

Ultralente insulin: is a long-acting insulin. On average, ultralente insulin starts to lower blood glucose within four to six hours after injection. It has its strongest effect ten to eighteen hours after injection but keeps working 24–28 hours after injection.

Unit of insulin: is the basic measure of insulin. U-100 insulin means 100 units of insulin per millilitre (ml) or cubic centimetre (cc) of solution.

Urea: is a waste product found in the blood that results from the normal breakdown of protein in the liver. Urea is normally removed from the blood by the kidneys and then excreted in the urine.

Uremia: is the illness associated with the build-up of urea in the blood because the kidneys are not working effectively. Symptoms include nausea, vomiting, loss of appetite, weakness, and mental confusion.

Urine: is the liquid waste product filtered from the blood by the kidneys, stored in the bladder, and expelled from the body by the act of urinating.

Urine testing: is also called urinalysis. It is a test of a urine sample to diagnose diseases of the urinary system and other body systems. Urine may also be checked for signs of bleeding. Some tests use a single urine sample. For others, a 24-hour collection may be needed. Sometimes a sample is 'cultured' to see exactly what type of bacteria grows.

Urologist: is a doctor who treats people who have urinary tract problems. A urologist also cares for men who have problems with their genital organs, such as impotence.

V

Varicose veins: are abnormally enlarged superficial veins mainly in the legs. They may be due to a weakness in the walls of the superficial veins, causing the veins to lose their elasticity and to stretch.

Vascular: is a term indicating the body's blood vessels.

Vein: is a blood vessel that carries blood to the heart.

Very-long-acting insulin: is a type of insulin that starts to lower blood glucose within one hour after injection and keeps working evenly for 24 hours after injection.

Very-low-density lipoprotein (VLDL) cholesterol: is a form of cholesterol in the blood. High levels of VLDL may be related to cardiovascular disease.

Vitrectomy: is the surgery performed to restore sight in which the surgeon removes the cloudy vitreous humour in the eye and replaces it with a salt solution.

Vitreous humour: is the clear gel that lies behind the eye's lens and in front of the retina.

Void: to urinate; to empty the bladder.

W

Wound care: includes steps taken to ensure that a wound such as a foot ulcer heals correctly. People with diabetes need to take special precautions so that wounds do not become infected.

X

Xylitol: is a carbohydrate-based sweetener found in plants and used as a substitute for sugar; it provides calories. It is found in some mints and chewing gum.

50/50 insulin: is a pre-mixed insulin that is 50 per cent intermediate-acting (NPH) insulin and 50 per cent short-acting (regular) insulin.

70/30 insulin: is a pre-mixed insulin that is 70 per cent intermediate-acting (NPH) insulin and 30 per cent short-acting (regular) insulin.

Appendix A

Cheating Out

Having diabetes is hard enough. Trying to manage your blood sugar levels during the weekends, at parties, reunions, festivals, and weddings is sometimes harder. My diabetic patients often ask if they can have 'cheat days' when they can consume, albeit in moderation, one of their old favourite foods. Something they can tuck into without it doing too much harm to their blood glucose levels. It is indeed very hard for them when there is a special occasion and there is yummy but unhealthy food everywhere and they can only eat the salad. I tell them to indulge in moderation and then consume an additional amount of their spice mix. They have to remember that this does not give them 'carte blanche' to over indulge all the time. If you are not on the spice mix, have a teaspoon of cinnamon and fenugreek seed powder, increase your exercise activity, and carefully monitor your blood glucose level. This guide should help you:

1 cheese sandwich: 30 minutes brisk walking
1 mutton Frankie: 20 minutes cross trainer + 45 minutes brisk walking

Appendix A: Cheating Out

1 chicken burger: 30 minutes jogging
1 fried samosa: 25 minutes slope walking
1 serving sev puri: 30 minutes on the treadmill at an average speed of 5.5 km/hour
1 serving chaat: 1 game of tennis
A small packet of wafers: climb up 8 floors
1 bowl popcorn: 15 minutes skipping
1 small katori alu bhujia/fried farsaan: 2000 steps in the balcony
1 serving fried pakoras: 45 minutes cardio
1 batata wada: 30 minutes on the football field
1 serving mixed bhajia: 30 minutes zumba
1 serving chicken lollipop (4 pieces): 45 minutes on the cross trainer
2 slices pizza (veg): 25 minutes Bollywood dancing
2 slices pizza (non-veg): 35 minutes Bollywood dancing
1 chocolate brownie: 1 hour on the treadmill at an average speed of 6.5 km/hour
1 small scoop of vanilla ice cream: 40 laps in the swimming pool
1 piece of barfi: 30 minutes spot jogging
1 ras malai: 20 minutes cross trainer + 1 game of badminton
1 gulab jamun: 30 minutes jogging
1 slice of fruit cake: 100 jumping jacks
1 large peg of whisky: 1 hour brisk walk + 15 minutes spot jogging
1 pint of beer: 80 laps in the swimming pool
1 glass of wine: 1 game of squash
1 glass of iced tea: climb up 10 floors, climb down 5, and then go back to the 10th floor

It is important to test your blood glucose levels post exercise and post indulgence.

Appendix B

Your Health Record Chart

NOTES

Name	
DoB	
Height	
Weight	
Blood Group	
Emergency Contact	

HEALTHCARE TEAM

Member	Name	Number	Address	Notes
Family Doctor				
Endocrinologist				
Cardiologist				
Nephrologist				
Ophthalmologist				
Podiatrist				
Dentist				
Nutritionist				
Nurse				
Physiotherapist				
Exercise trainer				

MEDICATION LIST

Name	For	Time	Dosage

On Days You Feel Sick

Call your doctor immediately if any of the following happens to you:

- You feel too sick to eat your normal meals.
- You are unable to retain food for more than six hours.
- You have nausea, vomiting, and severe diarrhoea.
- You have lost 3 or more kgs in a few days of being sick.
- Your blood pressure is higher than 140/90 or lower than 100/60
- Your body temperature is over 101 degrees F.
- Your fasting blood glucose level is lower than 60 mg/dl or above 200 mg/dl.
- Your post-meal blood glucose level is lower than 80 mg/dl or above 300 mg/dl.
- You are passing large amounts of urine and are feeling dizzy.
- Your breath has a fruity or acetone odour.
- You have trouble breathing properly or have palpitations and clammy skin.
- You feel sleepy or can't think clearly in the middle of a work day.

If you feel drowsy, are listless, have a sinking feeling, can't speak coherently, or can't think clearly, have someone call your doctor or take you to the nearest hospital. Keep your doctor's name and telephone number with you at all times.

DOCTOR'S VISIT RECORD

Tests	Dates and Results				
FBS					
PPBS					
HbA1c					
Frustosamine					
Total Cholesterol					
HDL					
Non-HDL					
LDL					
VLDL					
Triglycerides					
CRP					
Homocysteine					
Creatinine					
BUN					
Uric acid					
SGOT					
SGPT					
GGTP					

Tests	Dates and Results			
Sodium				
Potassium				
Chlorides				
Apolipoprotein A1				
Apolipoprotein B				
Haemoglobin				
ESR				
Microalbumin				
Urine sugar				
Vit D				
Vit B12				

Appendix B: Your Health Record Chart Notes

Glucose Log Sheet for People Who Use Insulin

Daily Log

	Insulin Type	Breakfast Dose	Breakfast Blood Sugar	Lunch Dose	Lunch Blood Sugar	Dinner Dose	Dinner Blood Sugar	Bedtime Dose	Bedtime Blood Sugar	Other Dose	Other Blood Sugar	Notes
Mon												
Tues												
Wed												
Thurs												
Fri												
Sat												
Sun												

Appendix B: Your Health Record Chart Notes

Glucose Log Sheet for People Who Do Not Use Insulin

	Fasting	Post-breakfast	Post-lunch	Post-dinner	Bedtime	Random	Notes
Mon							
Tues							
Wed							
Thurs							
Fri							
Sat							
Sun							

Dietary Recall

	On rising	Breakfast	Mid-morning	Lunch	Mid-evening	Dinner	Bedtime	Water
Mon								
Tues								
Wed								
Thurs								
Fri								
Sat								
Sun								

Appendix B: Your Health Record Chart Notes

Exercise Log

	Type	Duration	Calories burned	Pulse rate	Blood sugar	Blood pressure	Notes
Mon							
Tues							
Wed							
Thurs							
Fri							
Sat							
Sun							

Acknowledgements

Thank you, God, for the many blessings you shower on me and my family. I am grateful for every new and healthy day we have.

They say 'It takes a village to create a book'. Well, in my case, it took a country! I would like to express my sincere and heartfelt gratitude to the many people who so kindly saw me through the writing of this book and getting it birthed.

Thank you Milee Ashwarya, Pallavi Narayan, and everyone at Random House India who offered words of encouragement, provided much needed support, goaded me on to meet deadlines, and assisted in editing, proofreading, designing, and publishing. Each and every one of you is critical to the success of my book.

Thank you, Dr G.D. Koppikar, for being my mentor and guide, for believing in me, and taking pride in my work. You are an excellent teacher and have always inspired and encouraged me to continue learning with an open and positive mind.

Thank you, Mr Naresh Goyal, for taking time off from your busy schedule to write the Foreword to this book. Your cheerful disposition and zest for life are inspirational.

Thanks to all my clients from different parts of the country who penned beautiful words of praise. I am humbled, overwhelmed, and teary-eyed. Thanks to those who chose not to comment—I understand and respect your decision.

I am fortunate to be married to a man who loves me without restrictions, trusts me without fear, wants me without demand, and accepts me for who I am. Thank you, Savio, for your love, support, and encouragement; for letting me be who God designed me to be! I love you more than you could ever imagine.

My greatest accomplishment, my greatest success, and also my greatest pride and joy are my daughters Charlyene and Savlyene. Thank you, Charlyene—without your help with the reference work and typing, this book would never have found its way to the publishers. Thank you, Savlyene, for making me laugh, running errands for me, and egging me on when I was ready to drop. Always remember that the love between a mother and her daughters is forever!

Siblings share a lot—childhood memories, private family jokes, family secrets, joys and sorrows, and, most importantly, grown-up dreams and aspirations. There can be no better friend than a sibling and I am blessed to have two—my brother Chelston and my sister Laraine. Thank you for always being there for me.

Eating right is vital to diabetes therapy. I wish to thank all my diabetic clients who have shared their frustrations, trials and tribulations, and, later on, their joys and success stories with me. They have enabled me to write a better book based on their experiences in living and dealing with this metabolic disorder.

Thank you, dear readers, and all those who follow my 'Good

Health Always' programme for your interest in my work, your accolades, and your brickbats. Your words of encouragement and also of criticism have been of immense help to me in my personal growth.

There are so many more people I wish I could thank at this point, but time restraints, space constraints, and, of course, my modesty compel me to stop right here, right now.

Stay blessed with good health ... always!

Charmaine

A Note on the Author

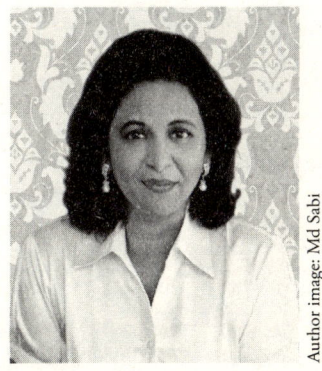

Charmaine D'Souza is a consultant nutritionist with more than 24 years experience in assisting clients who are interested in improving their health through better nutrition and natural care. Her vast and diverse network of clients includes celebrities and industrialists, all bound by the common cause of good health—the natural way.

In her first book, *Kitchen Clinic* (2013), Charmaine shared her secrets to good health—how to avoid minor ailments like colds, menstrual cramps, and headaches; control and prevent major illnesses like heart disease, and cancer; and stabilize diabetes. *Kitchen Clinic* is a comprehensive guide to herbal healing that can be done from the comfort of your home. *Blood Sugar and Spice: Living with Diabetes* is Charmaine's second book.

Charmaine lives in Mumbai with her husband and two daughters. She can be reached via email: goodhealthalways@outlook.com.